Designing Evidence-Based Public Health and Prevention Programs

Demonstrating that public health and prevention program development is as much art as science, this book brings together expert program developers to offer practical guidance and principles in developing effective behavior-change curricula.

Feinberg and the team of experienced contributors cover evidence-based programs addressing a range of physical, mental, and behavioral health problems, including ones targeting families, specific populations, and developmental stages. The contributors describe their own professional journeys and decisions in creating, refining, testing, and disseminating a range of programs and strategies. Readers will learn about selecting change-promoting targets based on existing research; developing and creating effective and engaging content; considering implementation and dissemination contexts in the development process; and revising, refining, expanding, abbreviating, and adapting a curriculum across multiple iterations.

Designing Evidence-Based Public Health and Prevention Programs is essential reading for prevention scientists, prevention practitioners, and program developers in community agencies. It also provides a unique resource for graduate students and postgraduates in family sciences, developmental psychology, clinical psychology, social work, education, nursing, public health, and counselling.

Mark E. Feinberg, Ph.D., is Research Professor in the Edna Bennett Pierce Prevention Research Center, College of Health and Human Development, The Pennsylvania State University.

Designing Evidence-Based Public Health and Prevention Programs

Expert Program Developers Explain the Science and Art

Edited by Mark E. Feinberg

Routledge
Taylor & Francis Group

NEW YORK AND LONDON

First published 2021
by Routledge
52 Vanderbilt Avenue, New York, NY 10017

and by Routledge
2 Park Square, Milton Park, Abingdon, Oxon, OX14 4RN

Routledge is an imprint of the Taylor & Francis Group, an informa business

Library of Congress Cataloging-in-Publication Data
A catalog record for this title has been requested

ISBN: 978-0-367-20514-0 (hbk)
ISBN: 978-0-367-20518-8 (pbk)
ISBN: 978-0-367-20517-1 (ebk)

Typeset in Garamond
by Deanta Global Publishing Services, Chennai, India

In all endeavors, I am grateful for the values I learned and lifelong support of my parents, Edward and Harriet Feinberg.

My own life and work on the art and science of promoting health and well-being is inspired by the creativity and wisdom of my children—Talia, Noam, and Shira. Each one is trailblazing a unique approach to leading a healthy and happy life based on curiosity, passion, and compassion for self and others.

Mark E. Feinberg

Contents

Chapter 1

Introduction

Mark E. Feinberg

Having completed training in theoretical, empirical, and clinical psychology, I set out into the world with a Ph.D. and a set of clinical skills that—hopefully—allowed me to help clients make positive changes toward better mental and behavioral health. Along with other new clinicians from counseling, social work, psychology, psychiatric, and other training programs, I had tried to develop better therapeutic skills such as listening, exploring emotions, reframing cognitions, supporting problem-solving, and enhancing behavioral control (along with case management skills such as case conceptualization, assessment, diagnosis, and treatment planning). But once I began working in the prevention and public health research world and developing new interventions, it became clear that my graduate training had not fostered skills for developing prevention and behavioral-change program curricula. And such skills were not anything I had sought out—in fact, until I began looking for my first job, I did not know that there was a field of prevention science in which program development was a key focus.

As I began developing a preventive intervention program for families, Family Foundations, I relied on my clinical skills and my theoretical understanding of behavior change principles in fleshing out actual program content. But a great deal of my curriculum development work was guided by my own personal experience and observation of others—what supports and catalysts had worked for me, what I had seen work for friends and family members in their journeys towards becoming mentally and emotionally healthy. Developing new program content, in that first project, and since then, began with brainstorming, and then proceeded largely guided by my intuition about what would work. More in the background than I want to admit, were empirically validated behavior change principles.

The subtitle of this book refers to the "art and science" of developing programs because, I believe, a great deal of the design of preventive and public health programs remains an art or craft. That is, whether we are trained clinicians or not, we bring our experience and understanding of how to facilitate positive, proactive change in ourselves, in other individuals, and perhaps in groups to bear in a creative process of developing new intervention models.

As scientists, we base intervention development as much as possible on the current knowledge base of risk and protective factors, mediating mechanisms, target population characteristics, and behavior change principles. Yet the actual construction of a preventive public health program consists of an active leap beyond our knowledge base. Similarly, an architect's design work is based on goals (how much floor space does a client desire, what loads must be supported, how many bathrooms are needed), informed by the knowledge of how different materials behave under different conditions. Yet the design of a new building emerges from a creative act that, while organizing building materials in ways that will facilitate the building requirements, is also concerned with shaping the experiences of people viewing or inside the building by creating an attractive, welcoming, stimulating, or comfortable environment. Although an architect's prior experience designing buildings informs the approaches taken to help shape such intangible experiences, a synthesizing, intuitive, and creative factor continues to be critical in developing new buildings...or behavior change programs.

For program developers from the research world, defining the risk/protective mechanisms affecting the outcome of interest based on existing research is the easy part. What is more difficult is, first, identifying a circumscribed target for change that is a lynchpin in the bio-psycho-behavioral-social system that leads to a cascade of positive consequences. Even more difficult is developing a feel for what supports, behaviors, and change mechanisms might be able to be taught to or conveyed to people that they will internalize and use in their life when challenged by internal or external factors.

The prevention architect's goal is to achieve the most good, for the most people, with the least amount of money and effort. Consequently, program content and approaches must work for people with a wide variety of attitudes, strengths, inclinations, experiences, and capacities.

A program developer then needs to develop a sense of what tools (thoughts, perspectives, or behaviors) might work to help modify targeted behaviors for the majority of people in the target population—and how to facilitate the learning, internalization, and deployment of those tools. Although much of this process depends on trial and error experimentation (e.g., piloting), developing an intuitive sense of what tools may work and how to convey them is invaluable.

The purpose of this volume is to convey the experiences of leading program developers focused on fostering mental, emotional, social, and behavioral health: How have they approached the craft and science of creating new prevention and public health programs? What factors and decisions were they addressing as they began their early work? What have they learned along the way? It is my hope that such accounts will convey a sense of the wide variety of approaches and trajectories that leading program developers have taken, responding to a felt need to address a range of concerns and issues across the prevention and public health spectrum. I hope these accounts will prove useful to students, trainees, interventionists, and researchers in developing the craft and science of program development.

In conceptualizing this volume, I was initially interested in the approaches taken by different program developers to the task of creating curriculum content. However, Matt Sanders suggested that my proposed focus was too narrow—that there are a range of processes and concerns that program developers must address beyond the development of behavior-change content itself. Agreeing with that, I widened the focus of the volume to include additional program factors that required attention and development, such as providing training, ensuring fidelity, managing intellectual property rights, the non-profit or business side of dissemination. Some authors focused on the task of content development, while others discussed a wider range of issues around program implementation, sustainability, and refinement. I believe that this mix reflects an interesting diversity of approaches, experiences, and interests of program developers that will be useful for those starting to develop their own programs.

I appreciate the contributions of all of the authors. Such sharing of experience and wisdom helps build a field, a body of knowledge, and the future strength and efficacy of future prevention programs. This also counters the tendency for academic incentives to halt collaboration. In academia, reputation, position, access to grant funding and so on is largely based on the quantity and quality of original, published work in peer-reviewed journals. To protect their intellectual capital, intervention developers sometimes shun collaboration, or collaborate only within their established team, limiting innovation and potential societal impact. Although maintaining boundaries around one's work is healthy, the trick is finding a balance between overly restrictive boundaries that shut down further innovation and allowing one's work to diffuse into the *zeitgeist* without careful testing and development.

A further pull away from collaboration and field-building is the lure of financial success if a program becomes valued and widely disseminated. I would venture that the economic value of effective and even cost-effective prevention and public health programs is rarely realized given the many challenges to the large-scale dissemination of evidence-based prevention and public health promotion programs. Financial issues can be complicated. An employee's institution—whether a university or non-profit research organization—typically owns all of the intellectual property that employee develops at work. For example, I own a small business that licenses the intellectual property of a program I developed at Penn State from the university in order to disseminate it; the business pays a royalty to the university based on sales of the program. But situations differ. I know of colleagues whose institutions declined to claim the intellectual property and instead gave ownership to the program developer because the program seemed to be of limited financial value compared to the costs of developing contracts and monitoring the IP.

For some—perhaps most—program developers I have talked with, starting and managing a small business in order to disseminate a program is a headache. Most researchers in our fields are not business oriented; we are not experts at, nor do we enjoy business activities.

A number of chapters in this volume discuss some of the challenges associated with dissemination, going towards scale, maintaining fidelity, and developing scalable infrastructure. Some programs in this volume—including the Incredible Years, Keepin' it Real, GenerationPMTO, Triple P, the Nurse-Family Partnership, Strengthening Families Program 10–14, Team Resilience and others—have had significant dissemination success. In some cases, this success has been due to a strategy for scaling up that program developers adopted early on and pursued with some degree of effort and devotion of resources. Other programs grew more slowly and organically, as awareness of the program's benefits spread among communities and decision-makers. The dissemination of other programs benefited from a large-scale government-funded initiative; and still others were fortunate to form a partnership with a national non-profit organization interested in promoting the program.

Some chapters in this volume describe programs that have developed a strong evidence base and are engaged in dissemination strategies that include translating the program for other populations and delivery modalities; for example, New Beginnings Program, the Anger Coping and Coping Power programs, and Familias Unidas have moved towards the development of web-based programming and delivery. Still other chapters in this volume describe programs that have only recently developed evidence and have not yet turned the corner towards achieving wider dissemination—Cod-Cod, SIBS, Recipe4Success. Accordingly, these chapters have a relatively greater focus on the nuts and bolts of content creation and refinement.

In the 18th and 19th centuries, public health pioneers were centrally concerned with reducing the transmission of infectious disease—as we are again today, as I write this in the early stages of the COVID-19 pandemic. The early public health pioneers veered away from older ideas about religious and moral causes of disease, and worked from a rudimentary understanding of disease focused on filth as a cause and transmission vector of disease. Public health efforts such as quarantine and isolation had often been initiated in response to intermittent epidemics; but in the "great sanitary awakening" of the 19th century, public health initiatives became proactive. Ongoing public health campaigns aimed to prevent disease outbreak through, for example, enhanced personal hygiene.

Early sanitary efforts were carried out on two levels: First, reformers encouraged changes to the urban built environment, such as incorporating channels and then sewers into street plans to carry human waste and refuse away from living areas. The goal was to reduce the "foul air" that was thought to convey and transmit disease. Second, reformers encouraged changes in individual behavior, such as hand washing. These two levels of work, the community and the individual, continue to define the basic approaches to public health and prevention today. The work described in this book is largely in the tradition of focusing on encouraging change at the individual level.

As descendants of the early public health and prevention advocates, we are likely addressing similar issues as they did as we design the interventions of the 21st century. What are the key behaviors to target to promote greater health and less suffering? How to frame a program's approach so that participants can see how the program is consonant with their own deeply held values and are motivated by an alignment of goals? How to sustain change? How to sustain the organizations and activities that create and sustain change?

As the public health and prevention fields have grown, impelled in part by a seemingly growing number of inter-related mental, behavioral, and physical health problems, opportunities for contributing to these fields have expanded. In addition to developing programs and conducting efficacy research, areas of work now include cultural adaptation and tailoring, methodological innovation, implementation science, cost-benefit analysis, and community-based participation. Each of these areas has become a field unto itself. As with the rest of science, public health and prevention science has increasingly become a team sport.

As I mentioned above, the pathway from initial program development to widespread scale up differs greatly across programs. Across these different trajectories, however, one common element among all of the programs in this volume is that the developers invested considerable time into establishing a rigorous research base validating the program's benefits. The science of replication has taught us that initial positive experimental results are often not replicated. Thus, dissemination has tended to await additional confirmatory trials, delaying dissemination over several years. Although this process can be painfully slow, it is the existence of a rigorous evidence base that has played a key role in the decisions by local schools or agencies, funders, and national policy-makers to invest in some of the programs described in this volume.

Unfortunately, new opportunities for our work seem to arise regularly. I have seen the emergence—or at least a new level of public recognition—of the importance of several new health problems over the past 20 years: new addictive substances such as prescription opioids, obesity, youth suicide, loneliness. As new social and health problems arise, some innovators move quickly to fill a gap and market programs or strategies that purport to address the new problem. For those of us committed to an evidence-based approach, these rapid responses may evoke a sense of jealousy, competition, or impatience in us at times. However, while others may more quickly gain attention and offer solutions, the slower path of piloting, efficacy testing, and effectiveness research leads to greater health benefits in the end. While there are important efforts to make our development and testing processes quicker, more nimble, and responsive, the need for careful assessment and replication cannot be bypassed.

For my own part, I have experienced impatience and jealousy at times when others achieve success with a program that has a limited or no evidence base. The advice I received from my primary mentor in prevention science, founding director of the Edna Bennett Prevention Research Center at Penn State, Mark Greenberg, has been helpful. Having developed PATHS, a leading social-emotional school-based program, Mark counseled me to keep my focus on doing good science. Pursuing high-quality, rigorous science in the interest of improving human wellbeing has been the core value of our center; and that is what, in the end, will prove most valuable. Over the years, I have developed a great appreciation for the lasting importance of our work when we do good science. Even if the programs I have developed or co-developed do not go to scale, I am content with having worked with other colleagues to illuminate how a new approach or strategy has potential to prevent and reduce suffering. Hopefully another developer will follow up on our work and move beyond it, achieving widespread dissemination after resolving the acceptability, implementation, or dissemination obstacles we have encountered.

In that vein, I hope this volume contributes to your own journey in integrating the art and science of developing public health and prevention programs. I encourage you to learn from the skills, perspectives, and advice offered here, and then develop even more effective and sophisticated ways of supporting health and well-being. Please then share your wisdom and knowledge with those who follow your lead, and help prepare them to contend with the new health and social problems that arise in their generation.

Mark Feinberg
Topanga, California

Part I

Child and Adolescent

Chapter 2

Cognitive-Behavioral Intervention for Aggressive Children

The Anger Coping and Coping Power Programs

John E. Lochman, Caroline L. Boxmeyer, Ansley T. Gilpin, and Nicole P. Powell

Starting Point

John Lochman's initial interest in working with children with behavioral problems started in his graduate school years at the University of Connecticut. His fellow graduate students and he were inspired by the prevailing enthusiasm for research-based behavior therapy interventions, and by emerging notions about community psychology, which emphasized how their knowledge of interventions could be taken into real-world community settings such as schools. These interests led two of the faculty, George Allen and Jack Chinsky, and two other graduate students, Howie Selinger and Steve Larcen, along with John, to implement an integrated, multilevel prevention approach in one school. His portion, considered to be tertiary prevention, involved a test of behavior-modification training that was delivered to teachers to use with their most problematic students. The results of all three of the program elements were encouraging, and this general framework for conceptually based school-focused intervention has served, relatively implicitly, as a basic foundation for much of his subsequent intervention research over the following four decades.

In the late 1970s Mike Nelson and John Lochman were on the faculty at the University of Texas Health Science at Dallas, working as psychologists in comprehensive pediatric health care clinics located within extremely low-income areas of Dallas. They received many referrals from the pediatricians and social workers of children with significant problems with aggressive behavior in their school and home settings. Mike and John decided to use their experience with cognitive interventions to create a cognitive-behavioral group-based intervention program for elementary school children. This Anger Control program was based on an anger arousal model and training approaches that incorporated both the self-instruction training methods from Meichenbaum and the social problem-solving training methods from Shure and Spivack. This anger arousal model followed from Novaco's theory that indicated that aversive, provocative events in the individuals' environment had no direct effect on their anger and subsequent behavior except as mediated by the individuals' appraisal of the events, their expectations, and their private speech. After initial pilot testing, the Anger Control program developed from its initial 12-session version into the 18-session Anger Coping program with the collaboration of several psychologists and counselors working in elementary schools in Durham, NC. Anger Coping was evaluated in a series of small, randomized control trials while John was on the faculty at Duke University Medical Center, demonstrating its effects in reducing observed and rated aggressive school behaviors. An NIH grant in the 1980s permitted an evaluation, across the accumulated small samples, of longer-term three-year follow-up effects of the Anger Coping program. Overall positive effects were found, but the results indicated that a subset of the children whose parents had received a brief behavioral parent training intervention in addition to Anger Coping for the children had the strongest reductions in problem behaviors (Lochman, 1992).

Given these results, Karen Wells and John collaborated to create a more comprehensive child intervention component (based on Anger Coping, but with almost twice as many sessions and additional content areas) which would be accompanied by a structured 16-session behavioral parent training program. This Coping Power program (Lochman & Wells, 2002) focused on more discrete social-cognitive and social processes.

Strategy and Theory of Change

Aggressive children were seen as having two primary areas of cognitive difficulty in this anger arousal model that served as the basis for the Anger Coping program (Lochman, Nelson & Sims, 1981). Children first had to accurately perceive and interpret the problematic social situations they encountered (aggressive children had cognitive distortions at this step, and were expected to have misperceptions and accompanying anger arousal), and develop methods for coping with their high level of arousal (self-statements; relaxation; attention-focusing). Then children had to go through a problem-solving sequence that involved thinking of possible solutions to the problem, considering the anticipated consequences of the solutions, and picking an optimal solution. Aggressive children had deficiencies in the number and types of solutions that they could generate, and focal problems in not anticipating the array of consequences they would likely experience following their behavioral choices. A prominent feature of this anger arousal model was that cognitions and physiological arousal related in reciprocal ways, requiring attention to emotional, cognitive, and behavioral dysregulation.

The Coping Power program's contextual social-cognitive model (Lochman & Wells, 2002) served as a basis for the parent component and allowed for changes in the child component. Social information processing models had evolved and expanded on the sequential series of cognitive processes that children display during their social problems. The Coping Power program child component thus included a focus on children's schematic expectations and social goals, on the automatic nature of the primary appraisal phase of these processes, on social perspective-taking, and on deviant peer influences. These social cognitive processing difficulties were found to be evident in both severely and moderately aggressive youth (Lochman & Dodge, 1994), but to vary in their relation to proactive versus reactive aggression, requiring attention to child-level characteristics during intervention delivery. These child-level cognitive distortions and deficiencies were recognized to occur in the context of, and partially due to, empirically-based risk factors in the child's genetic, autonomic arousal and executive functions, and to contextual risk factors in the child's family (parenting practices that involved low levels of positive parenting and high levels of harsh, inconsistent discipline), peer relations (e.g., rejection from most of peer group; involvement in smaller group of deviant peers), and community environment (e.g., disadvantaged neighborhoods with frequent violent crime). Within the family environment, the focus is on parenting practices that include both antecedent conditions (e.g., clarity of parental directions an instructions) and consequences (positive reinforcement; punishments), as well as factors that affect the parents' abilities to adequately interact with their children. Thus, there is attention to parental psychopathology, notably maternal depression, and marital/partner conflict.

Creating Content

In the initial development of the Anger Coping program, Mike Nelson and John integrated two intervention approaches that they had used clinically, and that they perceived addressed the frequently irritable-angry aggressiveness of the children who were referred to them. These two approaches also fit with their evolving conceptual model. In their graduate training years, John had experience with social problem-solving training, using the Spivack and Shure model (Spivack & Shure, 1974), and Mike had experience with stress-inoculation training (Finch, Nelson & Moss, 1993). They reasoned that it was important to first assist the aggressive children whom they saw to develop stronger emotional regulation skills, using a stress inoculation approach. Once children had some capacity to better regulate their arousal and to delay an automatic anger-based response for at least few seconds, then children's cognitive, planful problem-solving skills could be the focus of intervention. An operant procedure throughout the intervention involved children setting weekly behavioral goals, having those goals monitored by teachers or parents, and then receiving rewards for the points they earned. It was believed that this operant component was required to help these aggressive children begin to generalize the skills they were learning in sessions to real-world social situations with their peers, teachers, and parents. This integration of emotion regulation, cognitive problem-solving, and behavior modification work for aggressive children was a new direction for cognitive-behavioral intervention at that time.

The emotion regulation sessions in Anger Coping included a focus on emotion awareness and on emotion regulation. As a precursor to learning strategies for managing anger, they drew on the theoretical and clinical work of Novaco (1978). Children learned to describe various emotions in terms of associated physiological sensations, behaviors, and cognitions. Children viewed a brief video illustrating how a boy physiologically and behaviorally began to experience anger in a situation with his mother, noting his various body reactions that he perceived to be linked to his anger (e.g. sweating, knot in his stomach, rapid breathing). The boy in the video described his "angry thoughts" that sustained his anger, and then described several other thoughts that might reduce his anger (coping thoughts). Children in the intervention session discussed the video and applied these concepts to their own experience of anger. Once they became more adept at noticing their anger, children learned three "tools" for managing anger arousal, including the use of distraction (e.g., thinking of other favorite recent or planned activities), relaxation practices (e.g., abdominal breathing, progressive relaxation, guided imagery), and coping self-statements. Children participated in a number of graded exposure activities to practice managing anger arousal, drawing on their clinical experience and a paradigm designed to help children cope with teasing, developed by Goodwin and Mahoney (1975). First, they were exposed to lower-level anger triggers (e.g., mildly challenging games, role-plays involving indirect teasing, such as with puppets). After demonstrating proficiency at this level, they moved on to practice coping with higher-level anger triggers, such as direct teasing or conflict situations. Clinicians provided coaching to help each child develop proficiency in managing anger arousal.

In the key sessions on problem solving, children learned a step-wise approach to solving social problems effectively, drawn from Spivack and Shure's (1974) problem-solving model. These steps included: identifying the problem, recognizing my feelings, brainstorming a variety of options for how to solve the problem, anticipating the likely consequences of each solution, and evaluating the expected consequences of each solution and using this information to decide which solution to try first. During the brainstorming phase, children were encouraged to consider a range of potential solutions, including those likely to have negative as well as positive consequences. Groups were encouraged to generate their own slogan such as "Stop, Think, What Should I Do?" for their problem-solving steps. Children used these steps with current problems they experienced, and demonstrated their mastery by creating a group video illustrating effective social problem solving in action. The video typically included a problem stem, and then three choices, with at least one of those being deemed as likely to be competent and effective in that situation. Various members of the group played pre-planned roles in the video illustration. To develop the Coping Power Program, John Lochman, Karen Wells and Lisa Lenhart decided to make the child session plans more concrete and detailed, and then to add important new information about social information processing (SIP), evident in research at that time (e.g., Lochman & Dodge, 1994), which led the Coping Power Program to address additional SIP-related mechanisms. Thus, they wished to expand their focus on topics that they felt were underdeveloped in light of recent SIP research at that time, including addressing encoding and interpretation aspects (hostile attribution biases) of the children's initial appraisal of a problem situation, and addressing children's social and instrumental goals and schemas as they attempted to handle social problems. They also decided to follow a typical approach to each new unit in the program by first introducing the concept with enjoyable and non-threatening games and activities, then applying the concepts to problems in their lives, and then practising skills with role-play and video activities. The process of adapting and creating new content was a collaborative effort by John, Karen Wells and Lisa Lenhart. For the child sessions, they started with the existing Anger Coping program; John and Lisa then explored new ideas for activities from existing workbooks and discussions with counselors, and formally involved several school counselors and psychologists as consultants over one summer as they actually drafted and edited the content. The parent component sessions were largely drawn from Karen Wells's prior extensive experience with parent training.

The Coping Power child component added more extensive content about some topics already within Anger Coping, and then added some new elements to address mechanisms accounting for aggression and to create stronger child engagement in intervention. One example of an extension of an existing topic has been evident in their new sessions on emotion awareness. In addition to the prior activities, children also learnt to identify common trigger situations for specific feelings with structured activities (e.g., I often feel scared when I am alone in the dark). There is an initial focus on a wide range of emotions (e.g., happy, sad, excited, scared, angry). Then, increased focus is placed on the feeling of anger using a series of monitoring and practice activities. A thermometer worksheet is used to help children recognize the range of intensity of feelings. Children decide which labels to give to varying levels of a specific emotion (e.g., "annoyed" at the bottom of the anger thermometer, "mad" in the middle, "enraged" at the top). They then in subsequent sessions identify different triggers for different intensities of an emotion such as anger, and then identify coping tools they can use at different levels of anger arousal. Noticing the early signs of anger offers an important opportunity to manage angry feelings before they escalate to a level that is difficult to manage. To increase the generalization of children's use of their anger awareness and anger coping skills, children complete daily records of the intensity of anger experience, the triggers, and the coping method they used.

Another extension of session activities took place in the social problem-solving sessions, with the addition of game-like tasks, derived from their discussions with school counselors. In an activity illustrating the importance of persistence in problem-solving ("Blockers-and-Solvers"), children divided into two subgroups, with one being the Solvers and the other the Blockers. A problem situation was identified, and the Solvers identified a solution, then the Blockers found a way to make that solution not work. The Solvers then generated a new idea, and this sequence between Solvers and Blockers occurred for several more rounds, ending with a final solution from the Solvers. These activities were designed to introduce principles that were building blocks for problem-solving, but doing so in a fun, engaging, and non-threatening way, before they began to use the problem-solving model (PICC: Problem Identification, Choices, Consequences) with a variety of their actual problems with peers, parents, teachers, siblings, and others in their neighborhood or community.

The Coping Power child component also includes activities addressing new mechanisms that had not been directly targeted before, including organization and study skills (since many of their aggressive children also had problems academically), social perspective-taking, handling peer pressure, and using their interests and social skills to become involved in less-deviant peer groups. For example, the Coping Power unit on perspective-taking includes a series of games and activities that illustrate how a single stimulus can be perceived in numerous different ways, rather than only the first way that comes to mind. Activities developed in conjunction with discussions with school counselors include identifying alternate ways of perceiving common optical illusions, a freeze-frame role-play of a TV reporter interviewing several children involved in an ambiguous situation, and a "motive-in-the-hat" exercise where children attempt to guess the intentions behind a very brief role-play of an action. The primary focus in perspective-taking training with aggressive children is on encouraging children to recognize that it is sometimes hard to tell what others' motives were, and ultimately to consider alternative, less threatening perspectives in ambiguous social situations.

The Coping Power parent component addressed typical parent behavior training targets, such as enhancing positive parenting, introducing planned ignoring, improving directions, and presenting alternate consequences for children's negative behavior (privilege removal, work chores, time-out). In-session activities include discussion of the behavioral skills, followed by role-playing. Parents keep weekly records of their behavior tracking and reinforcement practices, and these are discussed in the following sessions. They felt that it was also important to address some of the issues that contribute to poor parenting, including parents' stress and distress. Thus they added sessions focusing on parents' stress management. Using a pie-chart to indicate how they spend time, parents discuss the many stressful events in their lives, and how that makes it difficult to spend time on reducing their own stress. Parents identify specific changes likely to help them feel less stressed and connect with their child in a calmer, more positive way. In addition, parents take part in deep breathing and active relaxation practices, and commit to regular self-care activities outside of their sessions. Three sessions near the end of Coping Power focus on family communication and problem-solving. Parents discuss how to maintain open communication and a positive relationship with their child, especially as the child becomes more independent.

Refining, Expanding, Disseminating

A series of randomized control efficacy studies have been conducted with the Anger Coping and Coping Power programs. Three years after intervention, boys who had received the Anger Coping (AC) program were compared with a group of untreated boys. The AC boys had lower rates of drug and alcohol involvement and had higher levels of self-esteem and social problem-solving skills. The AC boys were not significantly different from previously non-aggressive boys on these variables at follow-up. Although the overall intervention did not have longer term effects on classroom behavior, a subset of boys who also received booster sessions with parents did display lower rates of independently observed off-task behavior in the classroom. Based in part on these findings, the Coping Power Program was developed, and a series of randomized control trials have found that Coping Power can reduce boys' and girls' externalizing behaviors, substance use, and delinquency through one- and three-year follow-ups (e.g., Lochman & Wells, 2002; Lochman et al., 2014). The program has been designated as a promising program in lists of reviewed, empirically proven programs such as Blueprints For Healthy Youth Development, What Works Clearinghouse, and CrimeSolutions.gov. In the course of this programmatic series of efficacy studies they have found that it has been important, however, to move beyond simple efficacy research, and to explore how the program can be optimized through dissemination and adaptation research.

Adaptations that Refine and Expand the Reach of the Program

It is important for interventions to address children coming from diverse ethnic, cultural, and community backgrounds. Adaptations of the program can help to optimize its use for different populations and to enhance its effects on certain outcomes.

International Adaptations

Cognitive-behavioral interventions may be limited by cultural constraints, and thus need to be carefully adapted. Following a stepwise approach (Goldstein et al., 2012), Coping Power has been adapted for use in other countries. A Dutch version of the Coping Power Program produced greater reductions in overt aggression following treatment, and lower marijuana and tobacco use at a four-year follow-up, compared to children in the care-as-usual control condition. Adaptations of Coping Power have been tested in Canada, Italy, Pakistan, Sweden, and Puerto Rico, with greater reductions in conduct problems for children in the intervention conditions than in control conditions. These adaptations have ranged from concrete level translations of the program into a new language, to deeper level adaptations that have required changes to how material is presented. For example, in the Pakistani adaptation of the program, the manual was translated (into Urdu), and the cognitive and emotional skills were presented within the context of Islamic stories and practices (Mushtaq et al., 2017).

Internet Delivery and Intervention Length

One central structural barrier for utilization of mental health services is that intervention can be perceived by participants and practitioners to be too demanding and too lengthy. There are encouraging indications that briefer interventions can be effective. A briefer version of Coping Power (24 child sessions, 10 parent sessions) has produced significant reductions in teacher ratings of children's externalizing behaviors at longer term follow-ups (Lochman et al., 2014), similar to the effects for the full program. An innovative way of offering briefer interventions is to include internet-based content, making the intervention more accessible and efficient. Hybrid versions of existing manualized, evidence-based interventions such as Coping Power, that include much briefer versions of the programs carefully integrated with internet-based website activities, can be created (Lochman, Boxmeyer et al., 2017). A hybrid version of Coping Power's child component included 12 small group sessions (instead of the regular 34) and a website which included a brief animated and humorous cartoon series, *The Adventures of Captain Judgment*, developed to specifically illustrate Coping Power concepts and skills. Relative to a randomized control group, children receiving the hybrid program had lower rates of conduct problem behaviors than untreated control children. The use of technology can also enhance the cost-effectiveness of interventions. The hybrid version of Coping Power had a 60% reduction in the frequency of counselors' face-to-face meetings (a savings in cost of intervention of 44%) while still producing significant intervention effects on children's conduct problems.

Inclusion of Mindfulness Training

The Mindful Coping Power program was developed to maximize Coping Power's effects on children's emotional ability and reactive aggression. Led by Caroline Boxmeyer and Shari Miller, Mindful Coping Power is a novel adaptation of Coping Power in which mindfulness practices were integrated with the existing cognitive behavioral elements to more strongly reduce children's reactive aggression. Key mechanisms that have been associated with the development and maintenance of reactive aggressive behavior include reactive aggressive children's difficulty in encoding and attending to details in their social environment, intense bursts of emotional and autonomic arousal, rumination about provocations, and poor behavioral inhibition (Miller, Boxmeyer, Romero, Powell, Jones, & Lochman, in press). Because of the attentional and emotion regulation difficulties associated with reactive aggression, they anticipated that mindfulness activities (including noticing the present moment, pausing and breathing, use of yoga, and body scans) could be especially important in improving children's attentional control and capacity, and their emotional self regulation, by decreasing their experienced intensity of strong emotions and their capacity to recover from distress. All of the core content from the Coping Power child and parent components was retained in the Mindful Coping Power program. Mindfulness practices (Kabat-Zinn & Hachette, 2013) were integrated into Coping Power in three ways: (a) mindfulness-only sessions (several sessions were added to the Mindful Coping Power child and parent programs to introduce mindfulness theory and practice); (b) mindfulness in every session (each Mindful Coping Power child and parent session began and ended with a series of mindfulness practices, including the ringing of a chime, a breath awareness practice, yoga poses, and a compassion practice); and (c) integration of mindfulness into existing Coping Power activities (e.g., an existing component on identifying early physiological cues of anger was enhanced through regular body awareness practices; compassion practices informed activities designed to help children and parents see situations from others' perspectives; and thought awareness practices helped children and parents let angry thoughts "pass on by," and welcome other more compassionate thoughts). In a randomized comparative effectiveness trial, Mindful Coping Power yielded stronger effects than Coping Power on children's self-reported emotional, behavioral, and cognitive regulation and on children's stress physiology.

Adaptations for Parents of Younger Preschool Children in Head Start

The Coping Power parent program has also been adapted for use with parents of preschool children enrolled in Head Start, a federally funded preschool program for low-income families. This adaptation, Power PATH, was led by Ansley Gilpin, Caroline Boxmeyer, and Jason DeCaro, and was planned and completed in partnership with Head Start parents, teachers, and administrators in a truly integrated, two-generation delivery model. Children received the social-emotional curriculum at school (e.g., PATHS), while parents learned how to apply those lessons at home. Parents also learned self-care techniques to support their own mental health and parenting goals as well as the development of social support. In a five-year, ACF-funded, randomized controlled trial with 540 preschool children in Alabama followed through first grade, children who participated in the Power PATH program demonstrated reduced aggression and hyperactivity, improved pro-social behavior and emotion regulation, with parents reporting reduced distress and family chaos.

Adaptations for Older Middle School Students

Though effective interventions exist for addressing aggressive behavior in elementary school children, fewer such resources are available for middle school students. Yet the middle school years represent a critical time for intervention, as aggression that persists into early adolescence is likely to become more stable over time and is associated with antisocial and criminal behavior in adulthood. To address the need for middle school-specific programming, clinical researchers at the University of Alabama, the University of Virginia, and Johns Hopkins University collaborated to develop the Early Adolescent Coping Power (EACP). As an initial step, topic areas relevant to emerging adolescents were identified, including the growing importance of peer relationships, romantic relationships, more advanced communication skills (assertiveness, "I-statements"), cyberbullying, and social media use. Leader materials and student activities were developed around these issues and were integrated into the Coping Power curriculum. Developmental modifications were also made to existing content; for example, journaling was added to the opening review period of each session, and child-oriented activities were modified to be more age-appropriate (e.g., a basketball role play was substituted for a puppet activity).

Clinicians in Baltimore implemented the revised program with middle school students as part of a small pilot. They provided feedback on the program during weekly consultation calls, and modifications were made to address their observations, leading to new activities such as addressing how to repair damaged relationships and how to cope with cyberbullying. Once changes had been integrated into the curriculum, a second pilot was completed in three schools. Pilot data indicated that the program was feasible and acceptable, and that, overall, students responded well to the content and actively engaged in the program. A four-year, IES-funded, randomized controlled trial (Catherine Bradshaw, PI) followed, involving 720 seventh-grade students in Alabama and Maryland. One year follow-up data collection has recently been completed, with promising initial indications of intervention effects.

Dissemination

To be effectively used as a real-world intervention with behavior problem children in schools, it is essential that the program can be delivered by typical therapists, including, in the school setting, school counselors. The intensity of training has been found to be critically important in the use of Coping Power in school settings. In a dissemination trial, counselors from 57 elementary schools in Alabama were randomly assigned to one of three conditions: Coping Power-Intensive Training, Coping Power-Basic Training, or Care-as-Usual (Lochman et al., 2009). Counselors typically had master's degrees in counseling, and had little prior structured training in cognitive-behavioral manualized programs. In both training conditions, counselors received three days of training prior to the intervention as well as monthly consultations. The Intensive Training group also received performance feedback based on audio recordings of individual sessions. Training intensity was found to have a significant impact on outcomes, with the Coping Power-Intensive Training group showing significantly greater reductions in teacher-, parent-, and self-reported externalizing behaviors and greater improvements in social and academic behaviors than the other groups (Lochman et al., 2009). A follow-up study of this dissemination trial found that children with counselors who received the Coping Power-Intensive Training experienced smaller declines in language arts grades than children with counselors in the other groups after two years. This study indicated that with adequate training, regular school counselors could effectively deliver the program, and emphasized the importance of well-structured performance feedback during the training period.

Lessons Learned

Two of the primary lessons they learned had to do with the process of how the Coping Power was provided, and who provided it.

Format of Intervention Delivery: Group versus Individual

Because of concerns about possible limiting effects of working with aggressive children in small groups, due to the potential for peer reinforcement of deviant talk and actions, they decided to compare the usual group format of the Coping Power Program to an individual format, in conjunction with Tom Dishion (Lochman et al., 2015). Although the group format has produced positive outcome effects, they felt that the group format might be limiting the effect sizes, at least for some children. At a one-year follow up, at-risk aggressive children in both conditions exhibited reductions in externalizing and internalizing behaviors; however, the degree of improvement in teacher-reported outcomes was significantly more pronounced for children with lower levels of inhibitory control who received the individual version of the program (Lochman et al., 2015). Subsequent studies have found that children who had greater social orientation, using an oxytocin receptor gene as an intervention predictor, and children with greater emotional dysregulation, using pre-intervention autonomic nervous system functioning as predictors, also had better outcomes if seen individually rather than in groups. These results suggest that for some aggressive children, individual delivery of intervention is likely to be optimal.

Therapist factors

Given the concerns about group intervention for some children, they also decided to examine how therapist characteristics may affect outcomes in groups. Group leaders' clinical skills, evident in coders' ratings of leaders' warmth and lack of irritability during group sessions, were found to be predictive of greater reductions in externalizing outcomes at a one-year follow up (Lochman, Dishion et al., 2017). This finding about the positive long-term effects of therapists' positive and non-irritable behaviors in sessions is consistent with other Coping Power research. Counselors with more agreeable and conscientious traits are likely to deliver the intervention with greater quality and to sustain their use of the program in later years, and children working with therapists who have secure attachment styles have been found to have better outcomes. These findings suggest that careful and extensive screening and training of group leaders is necessary to limit potential deviant peer effects when group interventions with aggressive children are employed.

References

Finch, A. J., Jr., Nelson, W. M., III, & Moss, J. (1993). Stress inoculation for anger control in aggressive children. In A. J. Finch, Jr., W. M. Nelson, III & E. Ott (Eds.), *Cognitive behavioral procedures with children and adolescents: A practical guide*. Newton, MA: Allyn & Bacon.

Goldstein, N. E. S., Kemp, K. A., Leff, S. S., & Lochman, J. E. (2012). Guidelines for adapting manualized treatments for new target populations: A step-wise approach using anger management as a model. *Clinical Psychology: Science and Practice, 19*, 385–401.

Goodwin, S. F., & Mahoney, J. J. (1975). Modification of aggression through modeling: An experimental probe. *Journal of Behavior Therapy and Experimental Psychiatry, 6*(3), 200–202.

Kabat-Zinn, J., & Hachette, U. K. (2013). *Full catastrophe living (revised ed.): How to cope with stress, pain and illness using mindfulness meditation*. Oakland, CA: New Harbinger Publications.

Lochman, J. E. (1992). Cognitive-behavioral intervention with aggressive boys: Three-year follow-up and preventive effects. *Journal of Consulting and Clinical Psychology, 60*(3), 426–432.

Lochman, J. E., Baden, R. E., Boxmeyer, C. L., Powell, N. P., Qu, L., Salekin, K. L., & Windle, M. (2014). Does a booster intervention augment the preventive effects of an abbreviated version of the Coping Power Program for aggressive children? *Journal of Abnormal Child Psychology, 42*(3), 367–338.

Lochman, J. E., Boxmeyer, C. L., Jones, S., Qu, L., Ewoldsen, D., & Nelson, W. M. III. (2017). Testing the feasibility of a briefer school-based preventive intervention with aggressive children: A hybrid intervention with face-to-face and internet components. *Journal of School Psychology, 62*, 33–50.

Lochman, J. E., Boxmeyer, C. L., Powell, N., Qu, L., Wells, K., & Windle, M. (2009). Dissemination of the Coping Power program: Importance of intensity of counselor training. *Journal of Consulting and Clinical Psychology, 77*(3), 397–409.

Lochman, J. E., Dishion, T. J., Boxmeyer, C. L., Powell, N. P., & Qu, L. (2017). Variation in response to evidence-based group preventive intervention for disruptive behavior problems: A view from 938 coping power sessions. *Journal of Abnormal Child Psychology, 45*(7), 1271–1284.

Lochman, J. E., Dishion, T. J., Powell, N. P., Boxmeyer, C. L., Qu, L., & Sallee, M. (2015). Evidence-based preventive intervention for preadolescent aggressive children: One-year outcomes following randomization to group versus individual delivery. *Journal of Consulting and Clinical Psychology, 83*(4), 728–735.

Lochman, J. E., & Dodge, K. A. (1994). Social-cognitive processes of severely violent, moderately aggressive and nonaggressive boys. *Journal of Consulting and Clinical Psychology, 62*(2), 366–374.

Lochman, J. E., Nelson, N. W., III, & Sims, J. P. (1981). A cognitive behavioral program for use with aggressive children. *Journal of Clinical Child Psychology, 13*, 527–538.

Lochman, J. E., & Wells, K. C. (2002). Contextual social-cognitive mediators and child outcome: A test of the theoretical model in the Coping Power Program. *Development and Psychopathology, 14*(4), 945–967.

Miller, S., Boxmeyer, C. L., Romero, D., Powell, N. P., Jones, S., & Lochman, J. E. (in press). Theoretical model of Mindful Coping Power: Optimizing a cognitive behavioral program for high risk children and their parents by integrating mindfulness. *Clinical Child and Family Psychology Review*.

Mushtaq, A., Lochman, J. E., Tariq, P. N., & Sabih, F. (2017). Preliminary effectiveness study of Coping Power program for aggressive children in Pakistan. *Prevention Science, 18*(7), 762–777.

Novaco, R. W. (1978). Anger and coping with stress: Cognitive-behavioral intervention. In J. P. Foreyet & D. P. Rathjen (Eds.), *Cognitive Behavioral Therapy: Research and application* (pp.135–173). New York: Plenum Press.

Spivack, G., & Shure, M. B. (1974). *Social adjustment of young children: A cognitive approach to solving real-life problems*. San Francisco, CA: Jossey-Bass.

Chapter 3

Developing an Online Prevention Program

Lessons Learned During Creation of the Children of Divorce – Coping with Divorce (CoD-CoD) Program

Jesse L. Boring

Online programs are an increasingly popular way to disseminate prevention and intervention programs. They have a number of advantages that address some of the most serious obstacles to dissemination of manualized programs. Online programs also have a number of disadvantages that threaten their utility, particularly with regard to the low program completion rates common to them. This chapter reviews the creation, evaluation, and dissemination of an online prevention program for children of divorce: *Children of Divorce – Coping with Divorce (CoD-CoD)*. A clinical trial showed that CoD-CoD both reduced mental health problems in children of divorce and yielded unusually high program completion rates. Particular focus is placed on the process of transforming existing in-person manualized programs into an online format that maximizes the advantages and minimizes the disadvantages of online program delivery. I advocate a personalized approach to program creation capitalizing on the strengths of the scriptwriter and/or spokesperson. I also discuss a module structure used in CoD-CoD to increase engagement, participant success with home practice tasks, and program completion rates. The chapter concludes with a discussion of the lessons learned during the creation of CoD-CoD and suggestions for applying those lessons to the creation of future online programs.

Starting Point

Much like a living being, the Children of Divorce – Coping with Divorce (CoD-CoD) program developed through a combination of premeditated design (i.e., nature) and environmental circumstance (i.e., nurture). In graduate school I kept a notebook of stray thoughts and ideas for research that occurred to me while reading through my coursework. Examples include "Look at the cognitive impacts of using just medication for treatment," "Take non-responders from a treatment outcome study and test an alternative therapy vs. continuation of the ineffective one," and "Sign of busyness #2: Multitasking during sneezing." Since I had no particular project in mind when it came time to choose my dissertation topic, I went back through my notebook to see if it contained an idea that was both practicable and exciting. When I came to "Online video games as a vehicle for skills-based training," I immediately realized I wanted to create and evaluate an online skills-based prevention program.

When I began my Ph.D. program in clinical psychology, I dreamt of creating my own mental health program. As I learned more about the field, I realized how difficult it would be to find that opportunity. The moment I saw the idea in my notebook I realized my dissertation was my one, and perhaps only, chance to develop my own program. Creating an online prevention program married my three primary research interests of prevention, dissemination, and evidence-based treatments for children. I had a little experience creating websites, so I had (or thought I had) some sense of what it would take to create an online mental health prevention program.

In the first few years of my doctoral program, I became convinced that the field of prevention was at a critical point in its development. While there were many effective interventions (a number of which are discussed in this book), few of them achieved widespread usage due to the difficulties of dissemination. It was as though Jonas Salk had invented the polio vaccine without inventing a way to share it with the world. Online programs presented an under-utilized tool for addressing that shortcoming and I wanted to be a part of bringing them into wider usage. I was also excited about the idea of creating a project that was wholly mine. I have always been someone who is better off working 80 hours a week on something I am passionately interested in than working 40 hours a week on tasks assigned to me by someone else.

All of these factors led me to push forward with the idea of creating and evaluating an online prevention program. I had recently helped lead a long-standing social skills group for children with Autism Spectrum Disorder that was immensely popular in the community and, as a result, had a depressingly long waitlist. To address this issue, I initially wanted to create an online version of that program's curriculum. My advisor, to his credit and my immense gratitude, did not shoot down the idea despite having no interest in intervention research. He suggested I speak with Dr. Irwin Sandler at Arizona State University's REACH Institute.

When I spoke with Dr. Sandler my heart sank as he explained that he didn't feel comfortable helping me to create a social skills program. He went on to say he would be interested in advising me if I was willing to create a prevention program targeting children of divorce (an area in which he has decades of experience). My initial reaction was to resist this change, but I soon let go of my resistance and saw the situation for what it was: a stroke of luck. The part of the project that fascinated and invigorated me was not the target population; it was adapting and modifying the efficacious components of an evidence-based in-person program for delivery in an online format. By accepting the suggestion to focus on this new target population, I gained the benefit of the decades of experience that Irwin and his colleagues at the REACH Institute had in developing, administering, and evaluating programs for families experiencing divorce. This expertise, particularly in how to successfully recruit, administer, and evaluate a program with divorced populations, turned out to be essential to my project's success. One need only turn to the chapter by Dr. Sharlene Wolchik and Dr. Sandler in this book to get a sense of their impressive and well-developed program of research. Having access to this expertise was an enormous advantage for someone like myself who had absolutely no experience in program evaluation.

Strategy and Theory of Change

As I began conceiving of CoD-CoD, my top two priorities were to ensure that the program taught skills that would effectively improve the mental health of children of divorce and that these skills were presented in a way that encouraged youth to complete the program.

There was good evidence available for how to address the first priority. Research had identified four modifiable mediators of mental health in children of divorce (see Figure 3.1), and I decided to adopt these as the proximal targets of the CoD-CoD intervention. I also benefitted tremendously from reviewing three existing in-person, evidence-based programs for children experiencing family disruption: Children's Support Group (CSG) (Stolberg & Mahler, 1994), Children of Divorce Intervention Project (CODIP) (Pedro-Caroll & Albert Gillis, 1997), and the child component of the Family Bereavement Project (FBP) (Sandler et al., 2003). Though FBP was designed with parental bereavement in mind, its skills and activities were quite similar to CSG and CODIP and mapped neatly onto the mediators I wanted to influence. Pragmatically I also felt free to borrow from the FBP curriculum when creating CoD-CoD since Dr. Sandler was its co-creator and gave me permission to

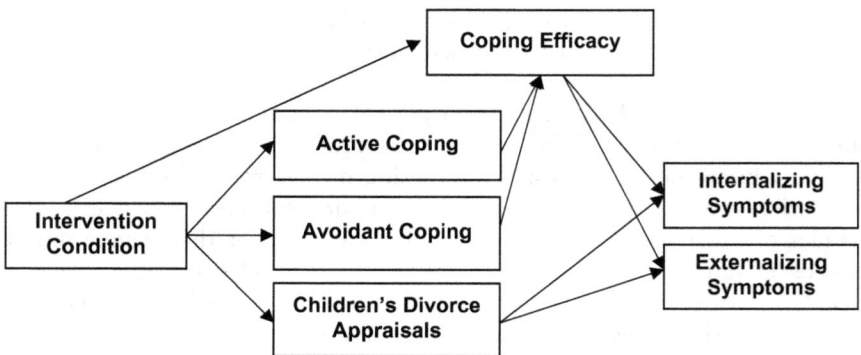

Figure 3.1 CoD-CoD Program Theory

do so. I had permission to review CSG and CODIP and this was helpful in identifying skills and activities that were common across the three programs. Since none of the evidence-based programs had research identifying which activities or skills produced positive changes, I had more confidence basing CoD-CoD on those they shared in common.

To distil the skills most useful to creating CoD-CoD, I developed a spreadsheet listing each activity of each program that identified if they addressed a mediator from my theory of the program (see Table 3.1). For example, I mapped activities teaching problem-solving skills onto the "Active Coping" mediator. I then gave each activity a score for its adaptability to an online context, usefulness in targeting the mediator, and entertainment value. I used these scores to filter out the activities that seemed to be the least helpful. Activities relying on group interactions were among those most often necessitating extensive modification. For example, FBP contains an activity where participants practice using their problem-solving skills by playing a problem-solving board game against other group members. In CoD-CoD I accomplished a similar goal by developing a game which participants navigate in a *Choose Your Own Adventure* style while using the program's problem-solving system to apply CoD-CoD's coping skills. The interaction they navigate is a realistic and challenging divorce-related scenario where one parent is criticizing the other. This game is built around video vignettes so that each choice the participant makes is followed by a video showing the results of their decision along with feedback on their choice. Wrong choices ultimately result in the opportunity to retry the failed scenario. The activity culminates in successful resolution of the situation.

I decided to split CoD-CoD into five modules with each module targeting one or more of the program's putative mediators. The first four modules each focus on developing a particular cluster of skills (e.g., Communication Tools).

Table 3.1 Skills Used to Target CoD-CoD's Mediators

CoD-CoD Skills	CoD-CoD Mediator
• Problem Solving • Positive Cognitions • Psycho-education	Increased Active Coping
• Feeling Awareness • Relaxation Training • Distraction Coping	Decreased Avoidant Coping
• Stressor Controllability • Reduced Wishful Thinking • Peer Testimonials • Coping Practice	Improved Coping Efficacy
• Positive Cognitions • Divorce Information	Healthier Divorce Appraisals

The final module fosters coping efficacy by providing opportunities to practice integrating those skills to solve problems and receive feedback on those attempts. For example, the final module contains an activity leading participants through addressing the three divorce related problems they identified as being most important to them in Module One of the program. With an overall program structure in place, I focused on how to successfully translate in-person activities to an online format.

In 2008, when I began developing CoD-CoD, few online programs had been created or tested. The emerging nature of the field presented an opportunity to innovate. I felt free to create the kind of program I thought would be appealing to the target age group and to let the outcome data determine the success of my approach. The disadvantage of this situation was that it meant there were few research findings that were useful for informing program creation. The finding from the literature on how to address engagement that seemed most relevant was that interactive programs are better at creating engagement than static programs (Barak et al., 2008). This was a helpful confirmation of my intuitions but was also so general that it provided little practical guidance for choosing among the possible approaches to creating an online program.

My background research identified a consistent pattern of online programs struggling to maintain engagement with users. Reported program completion rates were as low as 18.6% (Buller, Young, Fisher, & Maloy, 2006). This issue strongly influenced my approach to program development. I wanted to create a program that youth would be invested in returning to because it was useful, entertaining, and fostered a relationship between the user and the program. My approach to achieving these goals is discussed in the next sections of the chapter.

Creating Content

Translating In-Person Activities to an Online Format: Overall Approach

I was intent on minimizing the disadvantages and maximizing the advantages of online programs. My primary concern was the disadvantage of the impersonal nature of an online intervention. I worried it would be more difficult to foster engagement and program adherence without the social stimulation and pressures inherent in an in-person program. This disadvantage directly threatened my goal of maximizing program completion rates. As I thought more about the inherent impersonal nature of online programs I realized that paradoxically there was also an opportunity to be *more* personal. The narrator can reveal more personal information than would normally be advisable in a therapeutic relationship because of the one-way nature of the online interaction: The child does not have to manage their reaction to the narrator's personal disclosures.

Additionally, in a typical manualized program it would not be possible to script these disclosures into the program since by their nature manualized programs must be designed to be delivered with fidelity by any trained facilitator. Online programs however, can be delivered using the therapeutic strengths of the particular spokesperson since they are only delivered by that spokesperson and, apart from any technical glitches, the intervention will always be delivered with fidelity. This advantage, taken together with the fact that I would be serving as both the primary spokesperson and the narrator, meant I could script around my strengths. I took joy in the idea that I could apply my whole self to the creation of program content. I scripted skills I had such as playing guitar or riding a motorcycle into the introduction videos. I used stories of my own life, including experiences with my parents' divorce, to build a relationship with participants. I see this as a great and largely unrealized strength of online programs: They can capitalize on the individual strengths of the spokesperson in a way that is typically incompatible with a manualized program.

With an overall approach in mind and the basis for the skill-learning activities identified, I was ready to start scripting the program.

Scripting CoD-CoD

While drafting CoD-CoD's script I considered how to convert the spirit of each helpful activity on my spreadsheet to an online format. At times I was able to use FBP activities with relatively minor modifications for an online context. For example, sections of FBP where the group leader delivers information on coping skills in a monologue were easily converted to similar monologues with video or audio narration. One fairly typical example of the conversion process involved taking an activity from FBP where children were encouraged to identify which problems were theirs to solve and which were out of their control. In the original activity participants were shown a backpack with various objects with labels such as "Getting good grades," and "Family has no money." They were then shown that the backpack was a manageable weight if it only contained the problems a child could solve but became too heavy when it was loaded with all of the problems. In CoD-CoD this activity was turned into a video which began with a fairly faithful replication of the original activity. After adding textbooks with labels such as "Treating People Well" into the backpack I began to put in items representing issues the child could not resolve. This process included about eighty pounds of props culminating with a large cinder block labeled "Parent Sad A Lot." After placing the backpack on my back, I cut to video footage of myself trying to navigate various situations while wearing the heavy backpack (e.g., asking a girl on a date, playing basketball, and going swimming with friends). Needless to say, none of these scenarios ended well for me. This is an example of harnessing the advantages of an online program. I was able to demonstrate a wider variety of setting and scenarios where I would be hindered by the weight of the irresolvable problems because I was not performing the activity live. This video introduction was followed by an activity where participants were asked to sort potential divorce-related events into one of three categories: "My Job," "Not My Job," and "Gray Area." Participants then received feedback specific to each choice they made. The "Gray Area" category had not been a part of the original FBP program and is an example of using my intuition to alter an activity. I did this many times while creating the program. I felt comfortable doing so because I knew that ultimately the randomized trial would determine if the program was effective overall. I hoped, and still hope, to conduct follow-up studies to identify the exact elements that drive CoD-CoD's effectiveness. In this case, my intuition was that adding a "Gray Area" category for issues like "Mom says bad things about Dad," would make the program content more relevant for the participants and would provide a chance to think about how to use program skills in a real-world context. The strategy typically suggested for "Gray Area" issues was for the child to use their CoD-CoD communication skills to talk with their parents about the problem. If the parent was unwilling or unable to help resolve the problem, participants were instructed to use individual coping skills such as relaxation and positive cognitive restructuring to help manage their feelings about the issue.

As I wrote the script, I focused on individualizing the program to each child as much as possible in order to enhance participant engagement. I wanted participants to be able to choose the issues that were most important to them and to get feedback specific to those issues. For example, the online format prevented me from providing meaningful feedback to an open-ended question about divorce-related problems that participants experienced. Instead, I included an activity that asked the youth to choose the three problems most relevant to them from a list of 15 common divorce-related issues. CoD-CoD then provided feedback for each of the three choices which normalized these concerns and provided feedback based on children's typical experiences of divorce. Additionally, the participants' three choices were saved into the program's database. This information was then used in CoD-CoD's final session to guide participants in using program-related skills to address the issues they identified as most important.

Another design focus was to include game-like features in the program. Specifically, I was guided by the six gamification principles proposed by Garris, Ahlers, & Driskell (2002): Fantasy, Rules/Goals, Challenge, Sensory Stimuli, Mystery, and Control. For example, the Rules/Goals of a game are most conducive to performance when the game's goals are clear, specific, and difficult (Locke & Latham, 1990). To create this environment CoD-CoD used feedback via scoring and narration, provided performance based benefits,[1] and allowed participants to replay the game portions of the intervention. These features provide a design in which the overall goal is initially set at a difficult level while simultaneously encouraging persistence. This type of learning environment fosters the task mastery necessary for a skills-based intervention. CoD-CoD's program structure is designed such that each module adheres to the principle of providing clear, specific, and difficult rules. Whenever possible, individual activities within the program adhere to this same principle. A specific example of creating this type of environment occurs after participants learn CoD-CoD's problem-solving system and are asked to play a two-dimensional helicopter piloting video game. The game is quite difficult initially and the first flights commonly result in almost immediate failure: crashing. The youth are then led to apply their problem-solving skills to improving their performance. They are only able to continue on in the program once they successfully improve on their initial scores. Their scores are then placed on a high-score board and they are allowed to repeat the game as many times as they wish to improve their score.

The principle of Control was incorporated into the intervention by allowing participants to make choices determining the content presented to them (e.g., choosing which divorce-related feelings to hear more information about from among a long list of possibilities), directly controlling the video games at the completion of each module, and allowing the ability to navigate back to content or in-program games at any time. Providing these types of control is associated with greater motivation and learning (Cordova & Lepper, 1996).

I believe it is imperative to the success of CoD-CoD that participants use the skills they learned through the program in their real lives. This has been found to be true of in-person prevention programs (Schoenfelder et al., 2011). Application of the CoD-CoD program skills was encouraged through assigning home practice tasks at the end of each module. At the start of the next module, participants were asked about the previously assigned home practice. Four questions were asked: "Were you able to complete the home practice?" "How hard did you try to complete the home practice?" "How much did you want to complete the home practice?" and "Was the home practice helpful?" Users chose one of three responses to each question and were given feedback based on the exact constellation of their responses to the four questions. For example, if a participant reported that, even though they did not want to, they tried very hard to do the home practice, the feedback would acknowledge and praise their effort. A participant who was enthusiastic about doing the home practice but then didn't find it helpful could be reassured that with persistence the program skills would become easier to use successfully.

There was an inflection point early in the process of creating CoD-CoD when I decided to create the program exactly as I thought it should be designed, without concern for being conventional. I knew the data from the clinical trial would determine the success of my efforts. I resolved not to hesitate to include anything I believed would strengthen CoD-CoD. For example, when I was scripting an activity having to do with "hiding feelings," I decided to "put some skin in the game." Hiding feelings is a common problem for children of divorce as repressing feelings leads to a tendency to adopt ineffective avoidant coping strategies (e.g., trying not to think about the stressor). In order to illustrate the relief that often comes from disclosing difficult to share feelings I included a video of myself describing a situation from my childhood in which I wanted to hide my feelings about an issue that was trivial but extremely embarrassing. Specifically, when I laughed hard enough I would often pee my pants. I hid this (to the extent possible) from everyone in my life until my mid-20s. I was shocked at how quickly my shame became less powerful once I started sharing the issue with my brothers and then my friends. The issue quickly went from one which I found profoundly shaming to one which had little significance to me at all. It seemed like an ideal example of the power of opening up about hidden feelings and one likely to inspire a feeling of coping efficacy through vicarious modeling (Bandura, 1997). An additional benefit was that it sent a clear message to users that they were not just going through a generic program scripted by one person and presented by another. I believed CoD-CoD would come across as authentic since it was, in fact, authentic. It was unlike anything I had seen in other manualized programs. (It is not terribly difficult to imagine why that might be the case.)

As I developed scripts for the program, I seeded them with some of my real experiences. These included using formal problem-solving steps to make my way off a mountain I was stranded on, reactions to divorce-related events in my own life, being bullied by my siblings as a child, and stray observations I thought would be entertaining. I included videos starring my real family and friends, whom I introduced using their real names and relations to me. The intent was to feature real chemistry, not faked relationships like those typically found in programs with paid spokespeople and actors who do not know each other. I strove for the kind of wholeness of environment once eloquently described by singer-songwriter Tom Waits: "I think all songs should have weather in them. Names of towns and streets, and they should have a couple of sailors. I think those are just song prerequisites." My intuition was that creating a warm and authentic social environment comprised of multiple people the participants got to know better over time might be particularly appealing for children of divorce experiencing a significant family disruption.

The decision to take this organic approach was made much easier since as a graduate student with little external funding for my project a hi-tech approach was not an option. I recorded my narration on a cheap USB microphone I could plug into my computer and shot my videos on a digital camera duct-taped to a microphone stand. I did not see the low-budget nature of CoD-CoD as overly problematic. It fostered the creation of something rough and personal which is what I preferred. I was trying to create a YouTube channel, not network television. The animations in the program were done by amateurs I recruited from an online bulletin board devoted to making stick figure animations. An acquaintance at a summer camp I worked at while developing CoD-CoD became the female spokesperson/narrator for the program. I knew from watching her interact with her campers that her conversational style and sense of humor allowed her to easily develop a positive relationship with youth. I believe those same qualities allowed her to successfully build rapport with CoD-CoD participants.

Beta Testing

Once my first module was completed I began beta testing. I recruited my five step-siblings for the task. They had all experienced divorce and fell roughly within CoD-CoD's target age range. Possibly the most important thing I did during CoD-CoD's development was to sit near them while they went through the first module. They had questions and confusions that I had not anticipated. Controls that seemed intuitive to me were confusing to them. For example, initially the program had a button for moving to the next activity that was always active. This meant that the user could accidentally terminate an activity prematurely. My step-siblings clicked on buttons meant to be dragged (despite the audio instructions). They grew bored with long pieces of audio narration. Closely observing the beta-tests allowed for the resolution of the myriad specific problems with the first module's initial build and also revealed the general principle that navigating the program would always seem clearer to me than it was to users. I focused on making the controls intuitive and robust to different interaction styles. For particularly confusing activities I added animations demonstrating how the activity worked. As a failsafe, I also added redundancy when providing instructions by providing both audio and visual prompts to indicate what the user was expected to do.

Watching my step-siblings interact with the program and gathering other beta-testing data was also helpful in identifying the weakest parts of the program. For example, my step-siblings universally reported that the least interesting parts of CoD-CoD were the relatively long audio narration sequences. I was able to address this by shortening the audio clips and adding cartoon animations underscoring the points being discussed. My step-siblings enthusiastically embraced this change and some participants in the clinical trial reported that these animations were one their favorite parts of the program.

After pilot testing and revising the first module, I began scripting the other modules using the outline shown in Table 3.2 as the underlying structure for each module. (A comprehensive demonstration of CoD-CoD's module structure can be found at: http://familytransitions-ptw.com/CoDCoD/Sampl eModOut.php.)

Creating the Modules

While developing CoD-CoD I learned a deceptively simple truth about creating online programs: creating online programs requires coding. Psychologists

Table 3.2 The Structure Underlying CoD-CoD's Module

Activity Type	Purpose & Features
Home Practice Review	Provides individualized feedback (approximately 50 distinct possibilities) and social accountability around participant commitments to use programs skills during home practice.
Program Goal Check-In	Reminds participants of their program goal and provides feedback on progress that differs for each module. Shows participants a graphical representation of their self-reported progress toward their goal.
Introduction Video	Introduces skills to be learned while (hopefully) being entertaining. For example, one intro video was shot while the spokesperson (me) stood in the middle of a pond on a cold and snowy February day.
Module Content	The core of the program. Provides content related to developing the skills for each module using interactive activities, videos, animations, games, etc.[a]
Home Practice Selection	Users select a home practice activity requiring them to use program skills from the module (e.g., using communication skills to talk to a grown-up about a topic important to the participant).
Content Quiz	Reviews module content using 10 multiple-choice questions. The quizzes are designed to be difficult enough that achieving a perfect score requires careful attention to the module.
Reward Video Game	Each module concludes with a different video game. The games were simple but based on popular video game mechanics. In one game participants used computer keys to simulate playing guitar along with a song. In another they controlled a bouncing a ball in an effort to break all of the blocks on the screen. Participants used the score from their content quiz to buy advantages in the video games.

[a] Examples of CoD-CoD activities can be found at: http://familytransitions-ptw.com/CoDCoD/Sample2-10.php

are used to working in the medium of people and relationships. It is relatively natural for us to write a script to be delivered by people to other people. It is less natural to use computer code to deliver that content. I believe developing some proficiency at coding is crucial if you want to create online programs. I was forced to do this and I am glad I was. Without a budget for creating the program, I came up with the idea of partnering with a computer science student who would work on CoD-CoD as his senior capstone project. After creating the first module, the student worked with me as a contractor for the remainder of the project. However, I could not afford to pay him to work many hours, and it quickly became clear that I would need to develop some coding skills in order to help create activities and revise the initial programming. There is no quick and easy way to learn to code. Fortunately, I had the luxury of time since my dissertation was all I had to work on during this period in my life. I sat in the library for 10 to 12 hours a day learning to code using internet tutorials and (more often) trial and error as I attempted to apply what I was learning to creating the rest of CoD-CoD. Over time I gradually spent less time learning and more time coding. Learning to code—along with producing the narration and video content myself—allowed me a great deal of control over the finished product of CoD-CoD. It was also an efficient strategy: If I wanted to tweak the timing, text, audio, video, or look of an activity (this occurred literally thousands of times), I did so. I did not have to explain my thoughts and vision to a contractor and then evaluate and revise their work.

Refining, Expanding, Disseminating

Recruitment for Clinical Trial

Once the program was completed and revised it was time to recruit for the study. Based on a power analysis, I aimed for a sample of 150 participants to be evenly distributed to the control and intervention conditions. I attempted several different methods of recruitment including clinician referral, online advertising, email lists for school professionals, and meeting with school guidance counselors. After months of combining all of these methods I was able to recruit a total of two participants. This is a point where the expertise at the ASU Reach Institute saved the project. I eventually came upon a method, based on previous successful recruitment strategies employed at REACH, which actually worked: combing through court records to identify families with children in my targeted age range (ages 11 to 16) who recently filed for divorce. I sent a letter to each parent describing the study and the incentives for participation. The letter also explained that I would attempt a phone call to follow-up with them if the divorce records included a phone number. This method was laborious but dependable. I could reliably assume the number of children who would be enrolled in the study from this method would be about 5 to 10% of the initial letters sent out in each wave of recruiting. I sent out a total of 2,182 letters to potential participants. I then made 1,010 follow-up calls to these families. In this way I was able to enroll an additional 145 children over the course of six months.

Results of the Trial

The effects of CoD-CoD on mental health and preventing clinical problems from developing are documented elsewhere (Boring et al., 2015). One non-clinical outcome to note is that on average participants completed 76% of CoD-CoD with 69% of CoD-CoD participants completing the entire program. This represented the highest completion rate achieved in an online program targeting children up to that point. This is particularly noteworthy considering the difficulty that online programs have with program completion and the numerous novel strategies deployed in CoD-CoD to improve that rate. It seems reasonable to speculate that the engagement tactics such as using humor, dynamic feedback, individualized branching content, depicting authentic relationships, and the inclusion of genuine spokesperson disclosures may have been effective.

Dissemination Attempts

I created CoD-CoD in the naïve belief that if the results of the clinical trial were positive and I offered the program for free, it would be widely adopted. After two years of offering the program for free, I realized this would not happen. Not a single person used the program during those two years without me personally referring them.

I considered working with my doctoral institution (Arizona State University) to market the program or license it to a publishing company. However, such arrangements would lead to a loss of full creative control over the program.

I was able to retain ownership of CoD-CoD rather than the university owning the program; typically university resources are used in the creation of such a program which grants them ownership. However, I had developed the program working off-campus using all of my own equipment while living primarily off my student loans. I successfully contended that my dissertation topic was the clinical trial of the program, not the program itself.

Around the time I was becoming convinced that offering CoD-CoD for free was not a viable dissemination strategy, my advisor's company, *Family Transitions – Programs That Work*, approached me about offering CoD-CoD as part of their portfolio of programs. This partnership allowed an investment in advertising and the creation of a commercial portal selling enrollment to the CoD-CoD program. This commercial infrastructure allowed us to form other marketing partnerships. In particular, our commercial partner *EducationPrograms.com* has been successful in disseminating the program using connections to court systems which have chosen to offer or to mandate CoD-CoD in some divorce cases. Finding time to work on distribution myself has been challenging. Typical grant opportunities are not geared toward marketing or updating an existing program, and my position as an associate professor at a community college makes finding time to work on marketing CoD-CoD difficult. If you are an academic wishing to distribute an online program, I strongly recommend you find someone to work with who is passionate about marketing and has access to your desired market.

Lessons Learned

Test your program early and often—Testing your program on users outside of your development team is a critical part of the development process. Ideally this will occur early enough in the development process that it can influence the way you script your entire program. I highly recommend creating and testing the first module prior to scripting the remainder of the program. I used this approach with CoD-CoD and with every subsequent online program I have been a part of creating. This approach gives you a sense of the realities you will face in translating your ideas from the script to the screen. Having a more realistic and detailed understanding of your capabilities will allow you to script your program in a way that maximizes your capabilities and avoids liabilities. It is also likely to be much more efficient since it will reduce the amount of negotiation needed between those scripting the program and the coders tasked with implementing the script. I cannot emphasize enough the advantages of being firmly grounded in the realities of how your program will look and perform as early as possible in the scripting process. I suggest you budget time and money for at least three rounds of revision of the entire program including one internal review and two external reviews with your target audience.

The user interface (UI) is the foundation of your program—When I first developed CoD-CoD, I gave little thought to the way the users would move through the program. There was no clear indication when an activity had ended, and I had not provided users with controls allowing them to pause or replay audio narrations or to move backward in the modules. This setup was the result of an unexamined assumption that each user would understand every part of every activity the first time they experienced it, would never be interrupted, and would automatically understand when an activity came to a close. In later versions of CoD-CoD and in programs I have developed subsequently, I have focused on developing a more robust and user-friendly UI, including replay and pause buttons, activity titles and subtitles, and animations that use color and motion to indicate when and how to progress from section to section.

Build your program with the future in mind (but understand the costs)— Technology is constantly evolving and that can create headaches if you want your program to be continuously available. One of the most effective ways to make your program easy to upgrade is to place the majority of the code underlying the functionality of your individual activities in files shared between the activities. Coded this way, you can revise all of your activities by changing a code snippet in a single document that will automatically propagate throughout the rest of your program. This approach works extremely well for components of the program that you want to be uniform in look and functionality across all of your activities (for example, in the menu bar on the top of a page). The inherent cost to be aware of in using this method is that it makes customizing your activities (for example, so that each one is optimized for presenting the content you want to present) significantly harder. While developing individual code for each activity makes updating much more time consuming, it also makes customizing the activities much simpler. A hybrid approach in which some of the elements of each activity are taken from a common code document while others are written specifically for each activity is probably the best strategy in most cases.

Work with a developer who can do what you are asking of them—I have been the primary web developer on most of my projects but I have also used subcontractors. The primary criterion I use to select contractors is simple: Have they done a great job creating something similar to what I want them to create? This is true whether I am hiring narration talent, graphic designers, or computer coders; this is a critically important principle if you are hiring someone to be the primary software developer of your online program. Ideally when you look at the finished products the developer has created you will see how your vision can easily fit within the frameworks they have already made. By doing due diligence at this stage you will avoid a lot of problems and misunderstandings. Your developer will have already successfully dealt with many of the challenges and unwelcome surprises that come up when creating an online program. Be sure to ask the developer about the budgets for the projects they show you. Hiring a contractor to build your online program is like hiring a contractor to build your house. You are choosing quantity and quality at the same time so it is important to see how those two considerations are balanced in their work.

Write your scripts for the developers who will implement them—While you may think of your program as a cohesive whole, developers will think of your content in terms of the visual and component parts (e.g., audio narration files) they will use to assemble the whole. Including rough visual outlines in your scripts will help developers faithfully render your vision for the program.

Note

1   CoD-CoD modules culminate in participants completing a content quiz and using their quiz score to buy advantages in a subsequent video game.

References

Bandura, A. (1997). *Self-efficacy: The exercise of control*. London: Macmillan.

Barak, A., Hen, L., Boniel-Nissim, M., & Shapira, N. (2008). A comprehensive review and a meta-analysis of the effectiveness of internet-based psychotherapeutic interventions. *Journal of Technology in Human Services, 26*(2–4), 109–160.

Boring, J., Sandler, I., Tien, J., Crnic, K., & Horan, J. (2015). Children of divorce-coping with divorce program: Evaluating the efficacy of an Internet-based preventative intervention for children of divorce. *Journal of Consulting and Clinical Psychology, 83*, 999–1005.

Buller, D. B., Young, W. F., Fisher, K. H., & Maloy, J. A. (2006). The effect of endorsement by local opinion leaders and testimonials from teachers on the dissemination of a web-based smoking prevention program. *Health Education Research, 22*(5), 609–618.

Cordova, D. I., & Lepper, M. R. (1996). Intrinsic motivation and the process of learning: Beneficial effects of contextualization, personalization, and choice. *Journal of Educational Psychology, 88*(4), 715–730.

Garris, R., Ahlers, R., & Driskell, J. E. (2002). Games, motivation, and learning: A research and practice model. *Simulation and Gaming, 33*(4), 441–467.

Locke, E. A.,& Latham, G. P. (1990). *A theory of goal setting and task performance.* Englewood Cliffs, NJ: Prentice Hall.

Pedro-Carroll, J. L., & Alpert-Gillis, L. J. (1997). Preventive interventions for children of divorce: A developmental model for 5 and 6 year old children. *Journal of Primary Prevention, 18*(1), 5–23.

Sandler, I. N., Ayers, T. S., Wolchik, S. A., Tein, J.-Y., Kwok, O. M., Haine, R. A., … Griffin, W. A. (2003). The family bereavement program: Efficacy evaluation of a theory-based prevention program for parentally bereaved children and adolescents. *Journal of Consulting and Clinical Psychology, 71*(3), 587–600.

Schoenfelder, E. N., Sandler, I. N., Wolchik, S., & MacKinnon, D. (2011). Quality of social relationships and the development of depression in parentally-bereaved youth. *Journal of Youth and Adolescence, 40*(1), 85–96.

Stolberg, A. L., & Mahler, J. (1994). Enhancing treatment gains in a school-based intervention for children of divorce through skill training, parental involvement, and transfer procedures. *Journal of Consulting and Clinical Psychology, 62*(1), 147–156.

Chapter 4

Developing an Adolescent Substance Use Prevention Intervention

Keepin' it REAL

Michelle Miller-Day, Michael L. Hecht, and Jonathan Pettigrew

Starting Point

In 1986 Nancy Reagan, the First Lady of the United States, traveled to 65 cities in 33 states, raising awareness about the dangers of drugs and alcohol, coining the catch phrase heard everywhere, "Just Say No!" A plethora of "Just Say No" information campaigns surfaced in the media during the late 1980s, with most containing fear appeals (e.g., this is your brain—showing an egg: this is your brain on drugs—frying the egg in a smoldering skillet). Prevention messages recognizing the role of peer influence were phrased as "Just Say No" telling youth that it was a simple process to refuse the offer and that would suffice. By 1988 this program was ubiquitous, with more than 12,000 "Just Say No" clubs in the United States. Substance use and abuse in the United States was a significant social problem at that time—as it is now—and due to the attention given to the "Just Say No" campaign, federal support for drug prevention efforts increased significantly.

As scholars in the field of communication, Michelle (a graduate student at the time) and Michael (a professor) believed that this approach was too simplistic and that refusal skills (e.g., how to say "no") were fundamentally about competent interpersonal communication in the face of social influence. So, we joined forces to conduct basic research into the context of adolescent drug offers and refusals from the perspective of communication theory and research. At that time we had no plans for developing a program or translating our findings into something for future implementation. As scholars, we wanted to understand and explain problematic interpersonal communication in these contexts; that is, to understand the difficult task that teens face communicatively during adolescent drug offers—the who, what, where, and how of these situations.

Research literature on drug use cut across the academic domains of social psychology, public health, prevention science, and human communication. The basic premise of this literature was that social influence processes were central to peer pressure models of drug use, but as we explored this research in more detail it became clear that there was a gaping hole. Traditional social influence literature in psychology focused on the effects of various individual message characteristics (e.g., messages providing evidence or no evidence) and message sources (e.g., the credibility of the sender), and this research occurred almost exclusively in laboratories, divorced from *in situ* social interaction. The field of communication built on this earlier research and began to move toward understanding the message strategies involved in influencing others within the context of conversations. Instead of traditional research methods, such as showing participants a message and measuring responses, communication research focused on examining message strategies used within the context of the multiple "turns" occurring in an ongoing conversation. However, there was very little published literature in the early 1990s that studied these influence processes within conversations of importance such as drug offers, and nobody to our knowledge was capturing youth perspectives on drug offers, acceptance, and/or refusal.

Given these gaps in the communication and public health literature, first we sought to expand our knowledge about the social influence processes in drug offer contexts and then apply what we learned to the prevention of substance use, being careful to highlight the personal narratives of teenagers in our prevention efforts. The goal, in a sense, was to re-story or change the narrative surrounding substances, substance use, and substance users. Conceptually, this was an extension of the work Michelle was doing in the area of "trigger-scripting"—translating personal narratives into a dramatized presentation in order to "trigger" a reaction, heighten identification, foster understanding, prompt insight, and shift attitudes, opinions, and behaviors of audience members. We had applied this approach successfully in addressing issues of date rape, stepfamily conflict and communication, mother-daughter communication, and welfare-to-work social policies, work that was beginning to demonstrate the power of narrative persuasion. During this same time, Michael was describing effective and ineffective communication strategies in order to explain competent communication in problematic or difficult situations such as inter-ethnic communication and the disclosure of child abuse.

In order to identify effective persuasive narrative messages, we first described indigenous narratives—how youth were offering substances, what kinds of influence strategies were being used, and what youth were actually doing to resist these influence strategies. In the end, our approach—which endures even today—involves conducting interviews, collecting personal narratives, adapting those narratives into a performance script (often with the assistance of interviewees), producing public performances, and assessing outcomes. Inherent in applying personal narratives to developing prevention messages is the belief that health messages should reflect aspects of the target audience's experience and culture. Thus, the first step in our initial endeavor was to adequately identify the communication strategies that youth reported using when resisting offers of alcohol or other drugs. By listening to the narratives of youth about their own drug offer-resistance episodes, we hoped to identify how they understood the resistance strategies they employed and to learn more about how they perceived issues of substance use in their worlds. By doing so, we learned that—indeed—resistance is not as simple as "Just Say No."

We completed a series of basic research studies describing narrative accounts of adolescent drug offer processes (e.g., who offers and how the offers are made and resisted) with an emphasis on ethnicity and gender. This work spanned middle school, high school, and college-aged populations and was supplemented by survey research with large data sets. Our early research provided a descriptive basis for understanding adolescent substance use, and the social context of adolescent drug offers and refusals (Miller, Alberts, Hecht, Trost, & Krizek, 2000). This work revealed that youth primarily use four strategies to refuse drug offers: Refuse (simple no), Explain (no with an explanation), Avoid (verbal or non-verbally), or Leave. Since the early days of our research, detection of these strategies was replicated across age groups from childhood to young adulthood, and across the country and then the world. Identification of these strategies has even been replicated in resistance to sexual pressure.

After completing our initial basic research, we decided to develop an intervention to enhance teen's social and emotional competencies in the area of drug offers and refusals. This predated the current theoretical work on social emotional learning (SEL) but was similar in that the objective was to enhance early adolescents' social and emotional competencies including decision making, social awareness/refusal efficacy, emotion regulation, and relationships skills. Following the trigger-scripting approach developed previously, our first foray into intervention development was to adapt youth stories (narratives) of drug offers, resistance, and acceptance into performance scripts with two delivery modalities: live performance and video. These scripts were reviewed by groups of youth and drug prevention educators and revised based on this feedback. Once the scripts were complete, the live performances cast, rehearsed, and ready to perform, and the video produced and edited, we then conducted a group randomized trial of the intervention's efficacy. This early intervention was titled "Killing Time." Results indicated that both film and live performances were effective in decreasing self-reported use of drugs other than alcohol over a one-month period. This intervention, the process, and the performance scripts are described in greater detail in Appendix D of our first book (Miller et al., 2000).

During this work at the high school level, we began working more closely with prevention experts and learning more about prevention theory. This is when we realized that funding was typically geared toward prevention in early adolescence. The age of initiation for drug use was getting younger and the prevailing thought in prevention science was to try to reach youth right before they start experimenting. Therefore, we shifted our focus from a high school intervention to a middle school intervention. Additionally, the prevention field "encouraged" us in our grant reviews to consider a 10-lesson curriculum. Our basic research, the rich narratives collected across our studies, and the feedback we received from experts in prevention eventually culminated in the development of the middle school "keepin' it REAL" prevention intervention that is still used today.

The remainder of this chapter describes the strategic development of the middle school *keepin' it REAL: Refuse, Explain, Avoid, Leave* (kiR) program. kiR is a substance use prevention intervention comprised of 10, 50-minute lessons to enhance communication competence and social and emotional learning, teaching resistance skills, risk assessment, decision making, social support, and conflict resolution while targeting drug norms and expectancies. Recommended by the Surgeon General of the United States (2016) and several evidence-based program registries, the lessons can be taught by classroom teachers, counselors, after-school care, or community outreach personnel. A series of five student-produced videos forms the core of the curriculum based on narrative engagement theory. A "from kids, through kids, to kids" approach grounds the curriculum in actual youth experience, with media developed and produced by youth, and delivered to youth—who are then encouraged to develop their own prevention messages.

Theory of Change and Strategy

There were a number of theories that we developed alongside kiR, showcasing the interplay between theory development and practice. The following provides a succinct discussion of our overall conceptual framework and how the different theories influenced our program development.

Theories

The *Theory of Cultural Grounding* states that health messages should be grounded in the target culture, understanding and addressing its complexity and multiple identities. This theory points out that health messages will have the strongest influence when people see their group memberships reflected and acknowledged in the messages and argues that the active participation of cultural group members in message construction is a valuable strategy when making culturally grounded health interventions. This was accomplished by the research described above. Our original kiR was developed in Phoenix, AZ with a teen population that was largely Hispanic, Caucasian, and African-American. It also reflects gender/sex as a culture. Hence, the narratives reflected a teen culture through these ethnic lenses, creating "kid-centric" health messages.

Narrative engagement theory in its original form stated that conveying health messages through sharing personal stories and experiences can overcome resistance to the message, engage less involved audiences, reach low knowledge audiences, render complex information comprehensible, and allow us to ground health messages in cultural experience. Engagement in narrative messaging can lead to heightened cognitive arousal and empathy, reinforcing healthy narratives surrounding adolescent substance use, changing unhealthy narratives, and creating new mental models about how to think about substance use. Within our model, these culturally grounded narratives provide the foundation for shaping proximal beliefs, attitudes, and intentions that ultimately impact substance use.

Social emotional learning theory or SEL states that many different risky behaviors (e.g., substance use and bullying) can be prevented or reduced by improving skills such as understanding and managing emotions, improving communication competence, feeling and showing empathy for others, establishing and maintaining positive relationships, and making responsible decisions. The content of the kiR intervention was guided by the overall goal of improving the social and emotional competencies of adolescents through interactive lessons infused with culturally grounded youth narratives. These competencies are introduced, discussed, and practiced across the lessons with some lessons focusing on a particular competency while presenting skills for enacting these competencies. For example, in a lesson about communication and conflict, students increase their skill in verbalizing preferences that are not popular and understanding that a person can acknowledge another's views without necessarily agreeing with them. Refusal skills were central to the program, focusing four of the ten lessons on REAL (refuse, explain, avoid, and leave) competencies.

From Kids, through Kids, to Kids

The strategy for pulling all of these theoretical influences together into a cohesive intervention was to employ our "from kids, through kids, to kids" approach. Figure 4.1 illustrates this approach. *From kids* refers to gathering teens' personal narratives through interviews to reflect youth as well as ethnic culture, allowing youth to literally have a voice in the health messaging in each lesson. As indicated above, these culturally grounded narratives informed the development of the SEL program videos, role-play activities, lesson examples, and scenarios. Our process for creating this content is described in more detail below. *Through kids* refers to the community-based participatory research approach of involving youth in the development of the program

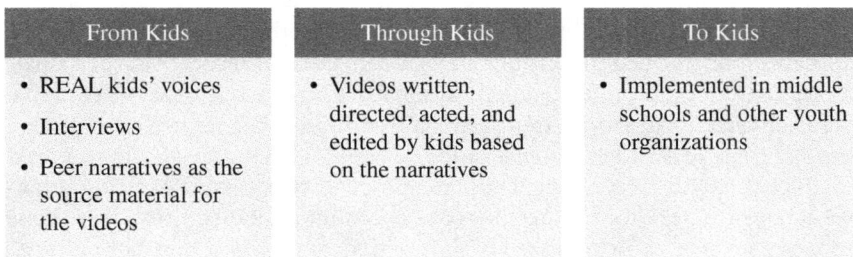

From Kids	Through Kids	To Kids
• REAL kids' voices • Interviews • Peer narratives as the source material for the videos	• Videos written, directed, acted, and edited by kids based on the narratives	• Implemented in middle schools and other youth organizations

Figure 4.1 "From kids, through kids, to kids" Strategy for Program Development

content as well as scripting, directing, and producing the kiR lesson videos that are central to the program, providing peer models for the resistance strategies of refuse, explain, avoid, and leave. Finally, *to kids* refers to implementation to early adolescents in both school and community settings.

Creating Content

Teamwork

The content of the 10-lesson intervention which includes a curriculum guide, presentation slides, lessons, student workbooks, and video production (five videos) was developed by applying techniques of community-based participatory research. This is a collaborative approach that equitably involves end-users and stakeholders as team members in the development process, recognizing the unique strengths that each brings. In developing kiR we included prevention researchers, youth, teachers, curriculum development experts, and school administrators in the process of development (e.g., content development and refinement, format, and design). A youth advisory board was recruited and came up with the name of the program "keepin' it REAL" in early 1996 to suggest a way of interacting in an authentic way that shows "who you really are." This broad team composition has been consistent over the years and has been employed in our various adaptations of the curricula. Involving administrators is essential for gaining access to other stakeholders to work on development teams.

Development Process

Our development process is illustrated in Figure 4.2 and remains the same after 19 years. This process involves six distinct phases (Colby, Hecht, Miller-Day, Krieger, Syvertsen, Graham, & Pettigrew, 2013).

Phase One

The first phase includes recruiting youth to share their stories of substance use offers and refusals. In a number of settings, we have sent college-aged researchers who are trained in qualitative interviewing to collect these stories. Young interviewers are trained to facilitate unique conversational spaces in their qualitative interviews to elicit detailed personal narratives from the adolescents. These conversational spaces are the arena where respondents feel safe to share stories of their personal experiences and life worlds (see Pezalla, Pettigrew, and Miller-Day, 2012, for a detailed explication of this process). Resulting narrative data can range from more to less nuanced and detailed, but all of these narratives serve to contextualize youth experiences within adolescent culture.

After collecting narrative data, we then conduct a thematic analysis and identify core resistance strategies and any other thematic elements to students'

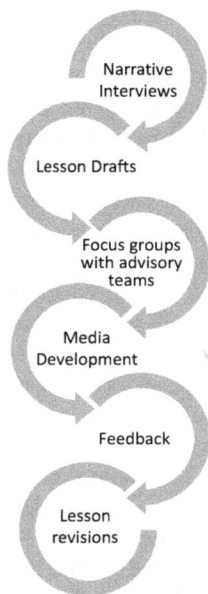

Figure 4.2 keepin' it REAL Prevention Intervention Development Process

stories. Combining prevention research theory and approaches (e.g., social modeling, resistance efficacy) with the findings from the interviews guided the content of our original 10 lessons. Theory provided the overall structure of the lessons, including: Options and choices, Risks and Consequences, Communication skills, Resistance Skills, Norms, Feelings (emotion management), and Social Support. Based on theory we knew that we needed to provide materials offering pro-social models and opportunities for skill practice to enhance self-efficacy. The narrative data helped us determine that there were four prototypical resistance skills (refuse, explain, avoid, and leave), and to promote resistance efficacy these skills needed to be taught in separate lessons. This resulted in our final 10-lesson format.

Narratives are integrated throughout the curriculum. They are used for examples or illustrations across curriculum lessons. For example, interviews informed classroom activities, vignettes, examples, and video scripts used in the lessons. Across the curriculum we sought to provide social models of effective refusal strategies, create opportunities for youth to practice skills, and challenge them to critically examine the effectiveness of strategies they could employ in a variety of social contexts.

For example, in the lesson specifically focused on the *avoid* strategy, interview excerpts provide examples of youth proactively avoiding (e.g., not going to the party in the first place) or reactively avoiding substance use (holding the red cup with ginger ale and pretending it is beer). A number of these stories from interviews were also adapted or combined into open-ended scenarios. The lesson places students in small groups and asks them to read these scenarios and imagine their responses, which they write in their lesson workbook. Small group work is included based on feedback from educators about the best ways to implement the activities and encourage interactivity, which is a hallmark of effective school-based prevention practice. Group work provides students with opportunities to engage in skill-practice with peers. The directions for one of these activities read: "Read the following scenario. Work together with your group to come up with three ways you could avoid this situation. Then decide with your group which is best way." In this activity there are a total of five different scenarios that youth discuss and react to in their workbooks. We use the workbooks to provide writing opportunities, give them a record of their responses, and reinforce the learning that occurred in the group discussion. These scenarios are all drawn from the narratives shared in the qualitative interviews. Additional "avoid" narratives are integrated into the program videos and other lesson activities. Lesson content is then reinforced through homework. For the avoid lesson, students are provided with a worksheet and asked: "Throughout the week take note of the times when you purposely avoid a situation or a person. In these boxes write what the situation was or who the person was, why you avoided, and how you avoided." At the end of phase one, all lessons are outlined—drawing content directly from the target population—with suggested activities, opportunities for practice, and homework. But this is just the start!

Phase Two

In phase two, we conduct focus group interviews with different adult stakeholders (e.g., teachers, prevention educators). In the focus group interviews, each lesson is discussed individually. Lesson outlines are provided, suggested content and activities are discussed. Valuable feedback is obtained at this point. For example, in our lesson about risks we pose a series of factual questions about adolescent substance use patterns derived from the Monitoring the Future Study of adolescent substance use (e.g., what percent of 8th grade students have ever smoked a cigarette?) (Johnston, 2005). We use questions to provoke critical thinking and to frame the content in terms of problems to be solved. Feedback from teachers in phase two suggested turning this set of questions into a think/pair/share activity. This was a great idea, but it was not until phase three that the interactive potential of this activity emerged.

Phase Three

In phase three youth and educator advisory groups review and provide feedback on the lessons. Using a cognitive interviewing approach (e.g., what are you thinking when you see that? read that?), advisory group members provide feedback on the lesson focus, content, activities, and homework. In our example from phase two, teachers had suggested a think/pair/share activity (dyads of youth get together and share ideas) for reviewing prevalence data and other statistics. However, the youth advisory participants gamified the activity resulting in "The Guessing Game." In this game, students are divided into teams of four to six students, and each team starts with 50 points. To win more points, the team needs to answer questions correctly. If the team answers the question incorrectly, they lose points. As part of the process, the team provides the answer they believe is correct along with the number of points they are willing to risk losing. Compared to where the activity started, as a series of factual questions, the approach that emerged through iterative feedback in phases two and three made the activity a better way to reinforce the concept of risk while imparting valuable information about substance use—as well as a lot of fun.

Phase Four

After the lessons are developed and refined by teachers and youth, the program videos are produced. These three to five minute films are scripted by teens (based on the narratives collected in phase one) and include the teens as actors in the films and as part of the production crew. These videos include student testimonials and brief dramatizations of effective refusal strategies drawn from the narrative interviews. The introductory video is part of lesson one and consists of an overview of Refuse, Explain, Avoid, and Leave, introducing students to the keepin' it REAL program. The refuse video is part of lesson 4, the explain video is part of lesson 5, the avoid video is part of lesson 6, and the leave video is part of lesson 7.

Producing the videos is exceptionally interesting and challenging. We are committed to keeping youth involved in the process, as reflected in our "from kids, through kids" approach. But we learned from our first experiences in collaborating with youth on video production that students are enamored with the possibility of using "fear appeals"—a persuasive message that attempts to arouse fear in order to increase caution and prevent harm. Unfortunately, persuasion research is clear that fear appeals are ineffective with this audience. First, there is no guarantee that an audience will experience fear rather than some other response (e.g., humor, revulsion). Consider, if you will, the infamous "fried egg" anti-drug messages that was intended scare youth about the physical effects of use but, instead, was turned into a joke. Second, even if the audience experiences fear, the extended parallel process model tells us we must effectively channel that response to achieve results. In prevention interventions the second step is difficult to achieve. Often fear appeals rely on an extrinsic force—a fear of punishment—that curtails unwanted behavior. Our prevention goal, however, is to develop an intrinsic desire—consideration of choices and consequences—that motivates behavior. This difference between teens' intuitive approach and research-guided strategies means that scripting the videos is often a challenge. Working with authentic source material (interviews) that needs to be adapted into a compelling presentation guided by prevention and persuasion theory is a sophisticated skill for anyone, so clear guidelines were needed early on to guide script development with youth. To address these challenges, during this phase of program development we hire a script writer to work collaboratively with the youth to identify the core stories they want to tell in each video, select narratives from our data that reflect the core stories in terms of characters, settings, plot, and action, and creatively integrate testimonial with dramatization to effectively illustrate and model effective resistance. One example stands out for us as both a challenge and advantage of involving youth. In our original videos developed in Phoenix, AZ the students were adamant about using—as one student called them—"real fake substances." To simulate smoking marijuana, they rolled oregano into a cigarette paper and simulated smoking in one of the films (which, by the way, demonstrated some styling break dance moves); however, the teachers insisted that this be taken out of the film. A compromise was made with students inserting a graphic in the final cut of film pointing to the joint with the word OREGANO! This satisfied all individuals. The conflict was between showing an illicit activity (negative modeling) and verisimilitude (having an authentic depiction of the youth experience). This issue of showing use has come up in all of the videos developed for this program (multicultural urban, rural, and international Spanish). In 2019 we produced new multicultural urban videos in Los Angeles with different youth who—again—wanted to use fear appeals and show "fake" use. But we were able to overcome these objections by showing them alternative messaging strategies early on in the scripting process.

Phase Five

In phase five, all lessons are completed, integrating the videos into each lesson. For example, in lessons with videos we add instructions for the implementers and also discussion questions for each video such as: how effective were the characters in refusing, explaining, avoiding, or leaving? Would you have used the same strategy in this situation? Why or why not? What would you have done differently? Questions help reinforce lesson goals by focusing students on the strategies being modeled in the videos as well as helping students project the modeled situations into their own experiences or imagined experiences. Having a discussion moves students away from focusing on the stylistic features of the video (e.g., clothing, accents, etc.) that might detract from its main objective. The content of the videos becomes an important guide for other lesson activities (e.g., role-play scenarios) that students are asked to complete.

Phase Six

In the final phase of this process, stakeholders provide feedback and suggestions for fine tuning the program content, format, and delivery. While this is the final phase before rollout of the program, it is far from the final feedback. Program development is an ongoing process with implementers sharing what has worked for them and what has not, and with the scientific community sharing new theoretical and practical discoveries. Although kiR is an evidence-based program and we are hesitant to make too many program adaptations, we have updated the original program over the years (e.g., removing references about pagers [!] and replacing those with references to smartphones) and, most recently, adding new videos and including vaping, social media, and sharing prescription medication in the lessons. Continual quality improvement requires attention to social, scientific, and educational developments and remains a key to effective prevention programing.

Refining, Expanding, and Disseminating

As kiR has expanded to new populations within and outside the United States, there have been changes to serve different audiences. We have adapted the program for rural Appalachian populations, for youth in Nicaragua, and for international dissemination with the D.A.R.E. organization. Each adaptation adhered to the six basic processes we outlined.

To illustrate how these processes worked out practically, we approached each adaptation with a sense of discovery. A hallmark of our process is learning from youth the who, what, when, where, and how of substance offers and responses (phase one). With rural and Nicaraguan youth, for example, we were determined to have an open mind, and reasoned that the regional cultures, social risk factors, and communal/familial resources in these contexts would look different from Phoenix, AZ, United States where the program originated. Specifically, the resistance strategies that these youth used might not fit with the REAL acronym. With rural youth, emphasizing a non-user identity ("I'm not a smoker") emerged as a potential resistance strategy. We eventually determined that identity was utilized as an explanation and as a type of proactive avoidance, but for a time considered that it might stand as its own unique strategy (i-REAL). Additionally, the settings and circumstances of the curriculum scenarios and examples would have to change. Approaching the adaptations as a collaborative endeavor with youth, educators, and local/cultural experts allowed for important modifications. Only after verifying what strategies youth used in these cultures, and to what effect, did we decide to maintain the REAL refusal strategies. In Nicaragua, because the program was translated into Spanish, the name also changed. We decided to call kiR *Dale, se REAL* which picks up on a common regional phrase and illustrates the two key acronyms used in the program. DALE is a decision-making acronym integrated across lessons and REAL represents the same four resistances strategies used in kiR which we discovered in narrative interviews with youth. A similar approach was taken when adapting kiR to create a sexual pressure resistance curriculum for adolescent Latinas. Interviews showed that in addition to refuse, explain, avoid, and leave, sexual pressure was met with more forceful or violent reactions (e.g., "I shoved him away!"). Identifying what teens actually reported doing in different situations allowed a point of entry for intervention and so sexual pressure was incorporated into this adaptation. The interviews were followed by curriculum adaptation for Nicaraguan youth. This was all done in collaboration with key stakeholders.

Fidelity and Training Considerations

Our experiences adapting the program (researcher adaptation) brought into focus the multiple opportunities for adaptation of program content and structure. Once the program began to be implemented, teachers were also positioned to make changes (i.e., implementer adaptation), sometimes benign and at other times more significant to the program. Recognizing that others have the power to adapt a program is an issue facing any broad dissemination. We were determined to empower teachers through training and ongoing coaching to best position kids for success. Rather than require strict adherence, we coached them during training sessions on the importance of implementation quality and encouraged them to only adapt when necessary. Based on numerous experiences working with teachers and other implementers, we hold an optimistic view that most teachers want to provide their students with the best chances for success in life. Although sometimes uninformed or misguided, teachers mostly tended to adapt programs to fit their own teaching styles, their students' experiences, their shared cultural context, and to accommodate practical time constraints (Miller-Day, Pettigrew, Hecht, Shin, Graham, & Krieger, 2013). In Nicaragua, where teachers' professional development opportunities are limited, they genuinely appreciated learning about classroom activities that engaged students in learning, discussion, and skill practice. Many found that certain class activities had utility in other courses they instructed beyond kiR. For these Nicaraguan teachers, we also repurposed observations of teacher implementation quality as opportunities for continued coaching toward successful and effective implementation. Following models of motivational interviewing, we highlighted and praised successful implementation practices and invited teachers to reflect on ways to improve in subsequent lessons.

Partnering

The most substantial partnership to date has been the dissemination of kiR through D.A.R.E. America. After several evaluations of their early interventions did not produce desired results, D.A.R.E. decided to view itself as a dissemination vehicle rather than a curriculum. After establishing a scientific advisory board, D.A.R.E. adopted kiR starting in 2006. D.A.R.E. is believed to be the largest provider of school-based prevention reaching 800,000 youth in the United States plus youth in 50 other countries. D.A.R.E. is taught by uniformed police officers who, despite 80 hours of rigorous training, still present a unique challenge in presenting prevention curricula. Officers are not trained in classroom management and their work often requires an authoritarian rather than participatory and interactive style of communication. In addition, D.A.R.E has a very complex constituency consisting of the national organization (especially its training staff and various boards), the officer-implementers, the students, state organizations, police chiefs/sheriffs, schools (including district personnel, principals, and teachers), the prevention community, and the media (who scrutinize D.A.R.E. closely and sometimes inaccurately). We collaborated on a process of "DARE-ification" that included adapting the lessons plans to D.A.R.E. format and terminology. D.A.R.E.'s keepin' it REAL curriculum was released in 2008, with the elementary school kiR released in 2013, and a high school curriculum in 2017.

We have argued elsewhere about the need for three types of adaptation: designer, implementer, and audience. Designers, we argue, should culturally ground and re-ground their curriculum. For example, D.A.R.E.'s version of keepin' it REAL has versions for urban, suburban, and rural cultures. Additionally, researchers show that implementers will inevitably adapt the curriculum (implementer adaptation). We try to build a curriculum that allows for some implementer adaptation while maintaining fidelity to core principles and contents (e.g., allowing implementer or student stories to fill in examples, providing individual, dyadic, and group options for activities, or utilizing discussion questions to localize and personalize content). Finally, we believe the audience members are not passive recipients of prevention content; rather they actively construct the experience for themselves and they interact in social circles that may or may not support the curriculum goals. Content should allow for some flexibility through activities and discussion that explicitly (e.g., planned moments of reflecting on and reacting to the lesson content) and implicitly acknowledge these processes (e.g., activities that include language such as "when you talk with your friends about this, what might they think or say?")

This partnership has been key to the international dissemination of kiR, and so maintaining a healthy partnership is essential. But it is not always easy. All organizations have layers of bureaucracy, and at times these layers can obfuscate our common mission—improving the lives of youth, families, and society. When everyone keeps their eye on that ball and the team includes competent individuals with character, it is possible to endure the (sometimes challenging) process of program development. Taking a humble view of teamwork in program development includes admitting that there are things academics can learn from implementers/practitioners and also ways that practice can be improved by academic knowledge. In Nicaragua and during rural adaptations, this involved liaisons who lived in various cities of implementation and had a pulse on the experiences of teachers across the regions where we worked. Liaisons functioned as part of the team, performed training, conducted teacher observations and coaching sessions, and kept the team abreast of new regional developments that might impact the program. Having a diverse team where members cohere around a common goal ultimately served the schools, teachers, and youth.

Lessons Learned

There have been many lessons learned over the years, not the least being the importance of involving end-users in the development process. However, to be honest, our biggest learning curve has been learning the business of prevention. We did not learn the basics of academic entrepreneurism in the academy. Nevertheless, the business of prevention is inextricable from the process of disseminating and implementing an evidence-based program to bring it to scale and to ensure sustainability. These goals are affected by myriad business decisions along the way. Some business issues that we found important are:

- Make sure that you submit to and list your evidence-based programs on evidence-based registries and clearinghouses. This is where end users typically look for programs to use.
- Build partnerships with groups that already have an infrastructure for dissemination. As academics, it is important to stay within our skill set and partner with others to use of different strengths and resources.
- Copyright or trademark your intellectual property.
- Brand your program and then market that brand.

Getting programs "out there" for others to use is, in the end, what we are all striving for in our research. A lot of work goes into this process. But in the end, we believe it is well worth the effort.

Referenes

Alberts, J. K., Hecht, M. L., Trost, M., & Krizek, R. L. (2000). *Adolescent relationships and drug use*. Mahwah, NJ: Lawrence Erlbaum Associates Publishing.

Colby, M., Hecht, M. L., Miller-Day, M., Krieger, J. L., Syvertsen, A. K., Graham, J. W., & Pettigrew, J. (2013). Adapting school-based substance use prevention curriculum through cultural grounding: A review and exemplar of adaptation processes for rural schools. *American Journal of Community Psychology*, 51(1–2), 190–205. doi: 10.1007/s10464-012-9524-8.

Johnston, L. (2005). *Monitoring the future: National survey results on drug use, 1975–2004 (Vol. 1)*. Washington, DC: National Institute on Drug Abuse, US Department of Health and Human Services, National Institutes of Health.

Miller-Day, M., Pettigrew, J., Hecht, M. L., Shin, Y., Graham, J., & Krieger, J. (2013). How prevention curricula are taught under real-world conditions: Types of and reasons for teacher curriculum adaptations. *Health Education*, 113(4), 324–344.

Pezalla, A. E., Pettigrew, J., & Miller-Day, M. (2012). Researching the researcheras-instrument: An exercise in interviewer self-reflexivity. *Qualitative Research*, 12(2), 165–185.

Part II

Parenting

Chapter 5

The Incredible Years Parent, Teacher and Child Programs: Foundations and Future

Carolyn Webster-Stratton

Innovation of Incredible Years: Where We Have Been and Where Do We Go From Here?

Starting Point

At this late stage in my career I am often asked:

> What prompted you to develop the Incredible Years (IY) programs 40 years ago? What was your motivation for the collaborative group and video mediated methods you used in your intervention programs to change parent, teacher, and child behaviors? Why did you choose a group collaborative approach over the traditional one-on-one approach? How did your research career come about?

As I look back now on my life journey, I confess there never was a master plan to become an academic professor, or to develop a business training others. Rather just the opposite, my primary goal was to become a better clinician to help families and children. The growth and development of the IY programs seems to have come about because of personal experiences, a particular passion, research studies, collective action, and ultimately a measure of serendipity.

Development of a Strategy and Theory of Change ~ Historical Roots

I believe that my love of children must have arisen from my 15 years of summers at a YMCA camp in Ontario, Canada both as a camper and then as a camp counselor. Modeling theory would also suggest that I was motivated to innovate and to bring about positive change in children's lives in part because my father was a model innovator, always working to make things better and accepting of the benefits of technology. In 1950, he filed a patent for the O'Cedar sponge mop that he designed so that people could stand while cleaning the floor, rather than be on their hands and knees. He encouraged my passion for photography, as I joined him in his dark room printing black and white photos from film and later processing pictures in Photoshop and printing in digital format. I have been told by my parents that even as a baby I was fascinated by observing people, as apparently, my favorite activity was being harnessed and tied up to the clothes line, or put in my pram outside (regardless of temperature) to watch people. As a teenager, I loved taking pictures of people and I currently still love sharing my narrated picture-heavy travel blogs with friends. Ultimately, my photography and video obsession resulted in my developing video-based intervention programs for parents, teachers, and children, evaluating treatment outcomes via video observations, and using video to give feedback regarding clinician intervention sessions and to assess trainer workshop effectiveness. My early experiences working in a dark room with film progressed to the editing and reproduction of digital video pictures via the computer, and taught me to expect change and to learn from it.

Several key mentors in my early 20s influenced my philosophy of helping others and my theory of how people might be motivated to change their habits. After completing my training as a nurse at the University of Toronto, I worked in Sierra Leona, Africa with an African physician. The goal for me was to train local people to help pregnant women eat healthier food and to breast feed rather than bottle feed in order to reduce malnutrition and mortality. While teaching women to eat more nutritious foods to increase their babies' birth weights seems like a goal that mothers would embrace, I found my advice was resisted or ignored. I had brought a generator with me so that I could show slides of people eating healthy foods and urinating in designated spots (so as to prevent schistosomiasis). This slide show in 1969 seemed like magic to the African people as they had not previously seen what photographic images came from cameras. So, while my teaching efforts did not change behavior, they did provide good entertainment and much laughter. Before long I learned that the reason these mothers did not eat much during pregnancy was because they did not want to have big babies that they could not deliver due to their own poor health history, including Rickets disease and flattened pelvises. Large babies were more likely to lead to serious tears and fistulas that could not be surgically fixed. I also learned that mothers bottle fed rather than breast fed because they believed powdered milk sent to them from America was the more modern way. Moreover, the idea of walking a mile from a rice field to urinate in a hole in order to prevent schistosomiasis was completely unrealistic. From this experience, I learned to ask parents about their own goals for their lives, to understand their individual circumstances and barriers, and to explore the reasons for their decisions. Moreover, a wise, African physician, son of the local chief, helped me understand the importance of respecting culture, community involvement, and being collaborative while integrating modern medicine and concepts alongside traditional approaches. He had set up a local board of 20 chiefs from nearby villages who would send out messages with some of my recommendations about healthy life style concepts, including the value of breast feeding, via drums (a precursor to emails).

Traditional African shamans were always included in helping treat patients alongside modern medicine. It became clear to me that the motivation for behavior change comes about not as a result of being told by others what to do, but from a collaborative, experiential, and culturally sensitive relationship amongst families, communities, and clinicians.

My subsequent Yale graduate school experiences—while becoming a pediatric nurse-practitioner (PNP) and obtaining a degree in public health—included a master's thesis for which I evaluated delivery of modern medicine to the Cree and Ojibwa First Nation people. I conducted this research while working as a nurse on an island in Hudson Bay, Ontario. The only non-native person on the island, I found that pregnant mothers were hiding for fear of being sent south by plane to deliver their babies in hospital. They preferred to have their babies in their own tents with familiar women around them; they were terrified of modern delivery rooms and the method of delivering babies with their legs held up in the air with stirrups. Subsequently I received a summer grant to interview Navajo women about their parenting methods and, post graduation, I worked for pediatricians offering parent groups and helping parents manage their children's behavior problems. After my marriage to a physician, we moved to Alaska where I worked for two years as a PNP with Tlingit, Haida, and Tsimshian people. Part of the time I was known as the "toy library lady" bringing in different toys on home visits to teach parents how to stimulate child development through play. I became convinced that "talking therapy" alone was not enough for parent behavior to change; I felt that change needed to be experiential, collaborative, culturally sensitive, and supported by a strong and trusting relationship with the clinician.

Dr. Kate Kogan was my third important mentor during my graduate doctoral studies in educational psychology. She had been trained by Connie Hanf (1973) to use the "bug-in-the-ear" video feedback and coaching methods with parents who had children with developmental delays. The "bug in the ear" method I learned included giving feedback to parents using edited videotapes of their interactions with their children. This was followed by asking parents to wear a small hearing aid while playing with their children. During my observations of this play time through a one-way mirror, I could give the parent in-the-moment clinical advice. For example, I could suggest replacing critical responses with positive responses, ignoring inappropriate behavior, and describing the child's actions rather than asking questions. Dr. Kogan's research outcomes with children who had developmental delays were compelling (Kogan & Gordon, 1975).

My volunteer work with Dr. Kogan re-ignited my earlier photographic passion. I was convinced that videotape and performance methods could be a more valuable therapeutic and teaching tool than the typical verbal cognitive approaches. I vividly recall the very first parent I worked with using video feedback. After showing her edited tape of her interactions with her child she started to cry. She said, "I have always seen my mother as very critical but have never seen the same behavior in myself." Seeing the video of herself set the stage for a self-reflective process of emotional release and behavior change. While I was entranced with the idea of using video feedback and bug-in-the ear coaching methods as a therapeutic tool with families, I realized that this personalized method was costly and time consuming, involving hours of editing, and would not meet the needs of the increasing numbers of parents wanting help managing their children's misbehaviors. I wondered if parents in a group format could learn from watching standardized videotape vignettes of other parents managing common behavior problems. There was considerable skepticism and disbelief that this group-based and collaborative parent approach—without the individualized bug-in-the-ear coached parent-child play sessions—would work to change parent behavior. Moreover, in the 1970s, most people thought I would never be able bring about change with this rarely used videotape modeling method!

To test my idea, for my doctoral research I developed a standardized video-based parent program with excerpts from the videos I had filmed from my bug-in-the-ear parent experiences. With this four-week, two-hour session program I conducted my first randomized control group study to evaluate the effectiveness of such an approach for improving parent-child interactions and reducing behavior problems. I hypothesized the parents would learn more through standardized videotape modeling, group discussion, peer support, and home practices with their children than from the more verbal-based one-on-one approach, which was considered the "gold standard" of parent training at that time. I believed that offering the program in the form of video vignettes designed to trigger self-reflection, group problem solving, and practices would be more cost effective and would provide often isolated and stigmatized parents with much needed support. I recruited parents of young children (ages three to six years) exhibiting disruptive behavior problems with the following short term goals: improve parent-child relationships, replace harsh discipline with proactive discipline, improve parent-teacher partnerships, and increase parent support. I hypothesized that targeting these parenting changes when children were young would lead to improved children's social competence, emotional regulation, school readiness, and prevention of social and emotional problems. The long-term goals were to prevent the development of conduct disorders, peer rejection, academic failure, delinquency, and substance use through the mechanism of teaching early effective parenting practices.

Creating Content

The basic parent content that was the underpinning of the video vignettes I developed for the first Incredible Years parent programs was based on the research and theory of the giants in the field of the 1970s. Gerald Patterson's work, including cognitive social learning theories about the development of antisocial behaviors in children (Patterson, Reid, & Dishion, 1992) was fundamental. His theory of change focused on interrupting negative, coercive parent-child cycles by teaching parents proactive discipline methods. The content that I developed related to children's developmental milestones was derived from Piaget's developmental cognitive stages and interactive learning methods (Piaget & Inhelder, 1962). The impetus for developing content aimed at building positive parent-child relationships was based on attachment theories (Ainsworth, 1974; Bowlby, 1980). A focus on building positive emotional relationships was not included at the time in standard behaviorally-focused parent training approaches. Finally, the basis of the cognitive strategies for challenging parent's angry and depressive self-talk, and the importance of developing support systems, came from Beck's research (1979) amongst others. I was lucky to be able to build on the shoulders of these amazing theoretical giants. I call this one of the serendipity factors in my professional development.

My first step was to take my theoretical understanding and put the IY content framework and sequence together. At the time there was some belief that parents should begin training by learning discipline (aka punishment) to manage their children's aggressive behavior because this was parents' primary goal. However, based on my earlier experiences, I felt that encouraging more positive parent-child interactions and relationships would be the necessary foundation for eventual behavior change. From Hanf's child-directed play concepts and my prior play therapy experiences, I developed a parent coaching technique known as "descriptive commenting", in which a parent describes a child's actions in real time—as if to a person who could not see the child. I taught parents to describe the specific positive behaviors that children displayed while playing, based on developmentally appropriate child behavior goals previously agreed upon with the parent. My theory was that this descriptive or narrated commenting was like enfolding the child in a warm, non-intrusive blanket of language that provided support to the child's play, showed the child that the parent was interested in them, and enhanced their language by linking words with the actual objects or actions. When children had language delays, parents focused on simple vocabulary words to expand children's language repertoire. When children had social skills deficits or difficulties with emotion regulation, parents described times when children were using positive social skills or were demonstrating regulation.

Over time I expanded descriptive commenting to include two other types of coaching that I called "social coaching" and "emotion coaching." Social coaching includes using descriptive language for the child's social behaviors: "You just shared those blocks with your sister," and emotion coaching includes describing the child's feelings, "You look so proud of your picture. I saw that you worked hard on it!" "Your sister looks happy that you shared with her." These two coaching methods extend beyond simple descriptive commenting and involve teaching parents to model and prompt social behaviors and emotional states in a non-directive way. Social and emotion modeling examples by the parent include: "I'm going to be your friend and share my cars with you." Or, "I'm feeling frustrated, but I'm going to take a deep breath and try again to put the puzzle together." Parent prompting children examples include: "If you want a turn, you can say: 'can I have a turn, please?'" or "I can see that you're angry. I bet you can stay calm and take a deep breath."

A few years later, after working with children with ADHD (about 40% of our sample of children with Oppositional Defiant Disorder also had elevated ADHD symptoms), I expanded the coaching methods further to include "persistence coaching." This approach was an effort to help parents understand how they could promote children's focus and ability to persist, stay calm and self-regulate when distracted or frustrated or bored. Parent persistent coaching examples include: "That's a hard problem, but you are really sticking with it." Or, "I can see that didn't work the first time you tried it, but you are staying patient and trying again to figure it out. I think you are going to figure it out."

With the addition of these highly refined coaching approaches, plus the addition of common strategies such as praise and rewards, my original four-session program designed for my dissertation expanded to a parent training course of nine two-hour sessions to cover this coaching based material. Today this child-directed and coaching material comprises the first 50% of the Incredible Years Basic Parent Program content. It seemed clear from the weekly session parent evaluations and initial outcomes that this foundational coaching and relationship work strengthened children's positive behaviors and self-regulation skills, replacing inappropriate, impulsive behaviors, reduced parents' use of negative or critical parenting, and enhanced parent-child attachment.

In subsequent years, I integrated my experience with fantasy play utilizing pretend characters and puppets within the coaching strategies, which led to even greater parent-child positive engagement. For example, a parent using a puppet could share with the child during play his feelings of sadness that his dog died, or disappointment his friend wouldn't play with him, or happiness he was learning to read in order to open up the opportunity for the child to talk about similar feelings. In some cases, children's conduct problems are a manifestation of single or multiple traumatic family life experiences. Parents' use of puppets or pretend characters to address trauma themes or life events similar to what their children may have experienced is a way to open up difficult communication. This tailoring lead to a trauma-informed approach to delivering the programs for particular populations.

Contrary to some parent programs available in the 1980s, I felt it was not necessary for parents to achieve "mastery" in the coaching methods or praise before moving on to strategies for directly decreasing negative child behaviors. The foundational relationship principles were continually referred to and strengthened further in subsequent sessions as part of the collaborative learning process.

The second half of the parent program content was focused on establishing consistent household rules, effective limit setting, and appropriate responses to misbehaviors. It was apparent from our interviews with parents that often they had no clear routines or rules and limits were either non-existent (permissive) or overly coercive and controlling (authoritarian). Based on the work of Baumrind on *authoritative parenting* (1966) and Patterson's "coercive theory" (1992), I felt it was important to help parents understand how to achieve a balance of clear and simple household rules and routines alongside nurturing and empathic responsiveness before teaching respectful discipline methods. I added strategies to manage misbehavior starting with the least intrusive methods such as distraction, redirection, and a planned ignoring approach.

I first learned about a "Time Out" procedure at a parent training workshop in the 1980s. That approach taught parents how to keep children who would not stay in Time Out by hitting them with a two-inch dowel rod. However, my Time Out approach was taught not as a punishment, nor were children ever restrained in Time Out, but instead was used as a respectful way to teach children how to calm down and self-regulate as well as to remove reinforcing (if negative) parent attention. Time Out was only used for children over the age of three and often required tailoring for children with developmental delays, ADHD, or with poor attachment with their caregiver. Children's developmental ability to understand and use the TO procedure is considered, as well as the importance of a foundational nurturing relationship as a basis for using Time Out.

Time Out was further refined to have children learn and practice how to take a Time Out to calm down before parents actually used it. This refinement came about after visiting a friend who wanted help disciplining her three boys who were constantly fighting. I was showing her the Time Out video vignettes and her boys came in and asked to watch. This resulted in a family discussion at a time when they were calm and receptive, followed by a spontaneous practice using Time Out to calm down. Later, when one of the boys hit his brother and was sent to Time Out, he went without resistance. I was convinced this worked well because of the prior teaching and practice of the procedure with the children. Subsequent to this unplanned personal experience, I incorporated teaching children how to take a Time Out to calm down as a standard part of our Time Out training for parents, teachers, and children. I developed new vignettes showing how parents can explain Time Out to calm down to their children (at times when they were calm) and then how to practice this with them using positive self-talk, deep breathing, positive imagery, and puppet practice.

The decision to incorporate beginning problem solving skills as the last program component for preschool and school age children (not for toddlers) was made to be sure that parents first had developed a positive relationship with their child as well as confidence in their limit setting and discipline approaches. When this is in place, children will already have developed some positive social skills and emotion management strategies so as to be able to engage in problem solving discussions and come up with possible appropriate solutions.

A decade later after delivering and researching the Child Dinosaur Curriculum, which heavily relied on therapists' use of large, child-size puppets (Wally Problem Solver), we began to incorporate more teaching of parents in how to use puppets, imaginary toy characters, and pretend play to model social skills such as helping, sharing, taking turns, waiting, and complimenting, to demonstrate empathy and emotional language, as well as how to use puppets to teach children calm down and problem solving strategies. Parents learned to use puppets to help children talk about feelings, practice self-regulation strategies such as deep breathing, positive imagery, positive self-talk, muscle relaxation, and managing traumatic situations. Even older children, who understand that puppets are not real, are still motivated to engage in this imaginary phase of cognitive development and enjoy playing being "detectives" and role-playing solutions to the drama stories involving hypothetical problems. About 10 years ago, I worked with a boy in our ADHD study who also had autism and had to be taken out of the child group because he was overstimulated by the noise and hyperactivity in the room. Interacting with this boy one-on-one with my Wally puppet helped me to discover that he had much more language, empathy, and social skills than I ever had observed in the child group. This convinced me of the importance of training parents in using puppets to connect with their children who had autism spectrum diagnoses as well as behavioral problems and ADHD. In fact, our recent work in the past three to four years with the autism parent program has resulted in expanding our BASIC program to include not only more puppet use and pretend play but also increased use of songs, nonverbal gestures, games, and visual prompts.

After I had my own children, I personally realized the impact of emotions and cognitions on parenting skills. There were times when I intellectually knew I should ignore my child's misbehavior but could not because of my emotional response and negative thoughts. Through my work with parents of children with conduct problems and ADHD, I became aware that content about appropriate parenting skills was necessary but not sufficient. Parents of these children were experiencing stress, marital discord, depression, isolation, poverty, trauma, and interpersonal problems that interfered with their ability to parent effectively. Almost a decade after developing the BASIC IY program, I developed the Advance program to address some of these additional risk factors, which as a supplement to the BASIC program led to significant improvements in parent and children's problem solving abilities (Webster-Stratton, 1994) and became one of the essential components of our treatment protocols for children with conduct problems and ADHD.

Video Vignette Development

The truth is that I developed the idea for a group video-based program from personal experiences, intuition, and a passion for photography, and subsequently searched for theories that would validate my methodological approach. Fortunately, the rationale for the collaborative, modeling, and self-reflective therapy methods I proposed could be found in Bandura's modeling and self-efficacy theory (Bandura, 1977, 1982). I designed the vignettes to trigger group reflective discussions, problem-solving, exploration of emotional and cognitive barriers, and coached practice. I discovered that video vignettes of parent-child interactions helped to normalize common parent traps, de-stigmatize a parent's sense of failure, and help parents be more empathic to children's individual viewpoints, developmental trajectories, and temperaments.

I began developing the child-directed play video materials in 1980 by filming hundreds of hours of parents and preschool children playing together. Originally I built a mock kitchen and living room studio set and filmed parents playing with their children with a series of toys I provided. There were no planned scripts as I understood from the theory of modeling that parents would be more likely to model parents who they perceived as natural, unrehearsed, and similar to themselves. I spent thousands of hours examining these tapes to find the 30-second to one-minute vignettes that illustrated a point about responsive, child-directed play. Here intuition and my gut reaction eventually determined my choice of over 300 video segments for the first parent program. I would describe this process as a bit like searching for love: You cannot exactly define what you are looking for, but you know it when you see it. Originally my programs had contrasting examples of effective and ineffective vignettes of parent-child interactions, but gradually I edited out many of the ineffective parent-child interaction strategies. I learned that the negative examples had a powerful and often dysregulating effect on parents, and were always the vignettes parents remembered the best. I wanted parents to have images of calm, patient, and loving parent-child interactions and not of yelling or criticizing children. Currently the more negative or less effective parent-child parenting vignettes in the programs are set up to allow parents to share and practice how to improve upon the interactions and to be compassionate toward the parent models.

In later years when our large expensive cameras with fourteen-inch reels of two-inch wide quad videotape film ($300 per one hour reel in 1980s dollars) became smaller, easier to use, and less expensive with the digital revolution, I was able to move the filming into parents' homes so that I could get more natural examples. For some programs I also was the second camera person who focused on close-ups while the professional would get the wide shots. I frequently knew where the camera should be before the professional did. In recent years, I added vignettes of parents or teachers talking about their

experiences participating in the IY program, which helped forecast participants' success if they continued to use the program strategies.

Once I had put together a set of vignettes that demonstrated a specific
concept such as emotion coaching, I then wrote narrations to precede each
set of vignettes. The narrations reviewed the main developmental, emotional,
or behavioral principle and primed the parents on what to watch for. I also
felt a summary narration would assure that the information parents got was
accurate and clear, and would prevent groups or IY group leaders going off on
tangents. In the leader manual I also suggested open-ended leader questions
to keep the discussion focused on the key learning principles for participants
to discover and subsequently apply to their individual goals.

IY Processes and Methods Development

Once I developed the vignettes and key content, my next learning process
focused on how clinicians could effectively utilize these vignettes to build
on parent strengths by inviting safe discussion, reflection, problem solving,
discovery of key principles, and setting up parents' individualized practice. In
other words, what were the important clinical methods and processes underlying fidelity delivery of a video-based program? This included how many
vignettes should be shown in one two-hour session; how much time should
be spent on video versus live modeling, and on cognitive discussions versus
practice exercises; how group leaders should handle parents' resistance to new
concepts; and how often a clinician should pause a video vignette to foster parent group discussions, self-reflection or trigger a practice exercise. What is the
correct program dosage and how will the intervention protocols be different
for prevention intervention versus treatment for children with diagnoses or
higher risk populations? How collaborative or prescriptive should the clinician leadership style be? When would confrontation or direct teaching be useful? How much attention should be given to changing parents' thoughts and
emotions or discussing past experiences versus targeted behaviors and future
goals? How can the group leader ensure training is culturally sensitive? How
are individual family needs and goals addressed alongside overall group process and learning? What adaptations are made to the program for less educated
parents, parents from different cultural backgrounds, or children with different developmental issues?

It became clear to me in watching hundreds of video hours of different
group leaders delivering the program over many years that, in addition to
group leaders having adequate social learning and child development knowledge, group leader relational characteristics (affect, warmth, humor, support,
leadership) and therapeutic and collaborative skills to promote the parent discovery process were key determinants of positive parent outcomes.

Each parent session starts with a "benefits-barriers" exercise in which parents discuss perceived positive reactions to the home activity or the new topic

of the day (for example, praise or ignoring), as well as any personal challenges or barriers that might get in the way of implementing the new skill. The discussions use a problem solving format: identifying the problem, identifying an alternative "positive opposite" behavior, practicing possible solutions, and reviewing barriers and how to overcome them. I believe these IY methods and processes are key to participants' ability to make meaningful changes. This understanding led to my writing a book for therapists about the collaborative process (2012).

How Research Affected Incredible Years Ongoing Program Development

Throughout my 35-year career at the university clinic, I continued to offer IY parent groups on a regular basis in the context of NIH-randomized control trials. Weekly session evaluations from parents, and video reviews of our sessions, as well as outcome data meant that I could find out what worked or did not work in comparison to wait-list control families. For example, one of my first studies focused on the value of using a video-based modeling group approach compared with the more personalized bug-in-the-ear approach. Once this research revealed that the video-based modeling group approach was as good as the one-on-one approach at post test, but provided more social support, was more cost efficient, and actually resulted in more sustained results at one-year follow-up (Webster-Stratton, 1984), I became committed to the group model as a core therapeutic IY approach.

Refining and Expanding

After 15 years of research exploring the best methods of training parents, it became clear that while the IY Parent programs could impact children's behavior at home, these changes at home did not necessarily generalize to classrooms or with peers. Consequently, the IY Teacher Classroom Management and Child Dinosaur programs were developed to see if the addition of one or both of these programs could bring about more sustained changes in children's behaviors across settings (http://www.incredibleyears.com/research-library/).

Over three decades of research, The Incredible Years Series has become a system of interlocking interventions that use similar cognitive, emotional, and behavioral clinical methods to include parents, teachers, and children. All focus on the same key outcomes, but act through different channels and with different developmental foci. All of the programs include the following methods: video and live modeling, group discussion and problem solving, short- and long-term goal setting, experiential practice exercises in the group and at home or in the classroom, promoting cognitive and emotional self-regulation and self-care, and building support networks. This learning occurs in a collaborative, reflective, and supportive atmosphere where teachers, parents, and children are encouraged to "discover" the solutions and builds on their strengths and experiences. The programs can be used independently, but research suggests that for diagnosed children and high-risk families, the effects are additive when used in combination. Each of the programs is thematically consistent, includes the same theoretical underpinnings, and is based on the developmental milestones for each age stage. There are a minimum number of sessions required but clinicians are encouraged to expand on the number of sessions according to group needs and background. The treatment protocols are longer than the prevention protocols in order to allow more time for individualization, enhanced practices, and showing more vignettes.

New DVDs, USBs and now some streaming of videos as well as group leader manuals have continued to be refined and created for different populations. For example, the parent program now has four different versions for distinct developmental ages from infants to preteens; I also developed a shorter, universal parent program designed for all parents of children of two to six years (Attentive Parenting), a program for day care providers and preschool teachers working with younger children (one to two and three to five years) (Incredible Beginnings), and two new programs for parents and teachers working with young children on the autism spectrum (two to five years).

Making the Decision to Disseminate ~ Challenges and Successes

Eighteen years after publication of my first study with the parent program and many positive randomized control group studies (Menting, 2013), requests began to come in for information about obtaining program materials and training possibilities. Largely these requests came from individuals in countries such as the UK, Norway, Denmark, New Zealand, and the Netherlands who had reviewed the research evidence and were interested in both evaluation of the program and dissemination in their own country, as well as researching their effectiveness for use in their population. I began an independent business to disseminate the programs. Because I had originally funded the filming, editing, and video production program costs with personal funds and not as a university employee, I retained full ownership, copyright, and trademark for the IY program. A contract with the university acknowledged this ownership, permitted me to use the programs for training and grant research, and stipulated that all further work related to marketing, training, and further product development would be done outside of the university. Until my retirement in 2011, I submitted financial disclosure forms yearly and participated in ongoing reviews regarding potential conflict of interest. A few years later, I decided to give up half my tenure salary and reduce my time at the university, spending the other half of my time engaged in disseminating the Incredible Years programs.

Having spent three decades as the developer of the Incredible Years series researching and expanding clinician manuals, video vignettes and protocols, I believed we had the tools to begin dissemination with fidelity. At that time, it was unclear to me whether clinicians would even need training because I believed everything was clearly articulated in the materials. However, I quickly learned from my video reviews of clinician group sessions than neither the materials nor brief workshops alone were sufficient to promote fidelity delivery. Clinicians needed help understanding how to tailor the discussions and learning to parents' and teachers' settings, goals, and cultural context as well as children's development level and diagnoses. A study of IY fidelity processes and strategies revealed the added benefits of ongoing coaching and support for clinicians as well as training agency administrators to support their group leaders (Webster-Stratton, Reid, & Marsenich, 2014). When I retired from the university, I pursued the dissemination journey in more depth by providing quality training, consultation, and ongoing support by certified coaches, mentors, and trainers, and promoting fidelity delivery of the programs through the certification/accreditation process.

Lessons Learned

As the developer of an evidence-based program (EBP), I did not understand that I would need to do more than develop the content and general procedures for program delivery and show positive research results. That was perhaps the easiest part. I found it was also necessary to develop a comprehensive training process, including ongoing support and consultation for the group leaders as well as for the administrators. The metaphor I use for developing and scaling up an EBP is building a house where there must be an architect (program developer) who takes advantage of changing technology and collaborates with the family or teacher around their needs and goals; a committed contractor who monitors building quality (agency or school administrator); onsite project managers to support and train staff (mentors and coaches); and a well-trained team of construction workers (group leaders). If there are problems in any of these links the building will not be sound. For example, when there are agency and clinician barriers, it is as if the contractors, hired electricians, and plumbers who were not certified, disregarded the architectural plan, and used poor quality, cheap materials. The Incredible Years Program Training Series has been set up with a supportive infrastructure of eight building blocks designed to promote program fidelity (Webster-Stratton & McCoy, 2015). The IY Series is now widely used in 18 countries; there are 8 accredited trainers, 75 mentors, and 110 peer coaches providing training and support to IY group leaders.

Lessons Learned and Next Steps

My experience has taught me that EBP development must be thought of as an ongoing building process rather than an endpoint. An important implication for prevention and dissemination science is understanding that effective programs continue to evolve and improve based on internal evaluation audits and feedback. As a parallel, consider that the safety features of cars continuously improve. Few people, when given the option, would opt to drive the old model without the proven safety additions. Gathering data on what works, eliciting ongoing feedback, and actively participating in the implementation of the intervention across a variety of contexts provides the needed information to improve interventions and meet the needs of culturally diverse populations.

Agencies charged with improving the well-being of children and families now have good options for selecting EBPs that are grounded in an extensive research base. The field has learned much about the necessary ingredients for successfully transporting efficacious practices into real world settings with diverse cultural populations. Some of the critical factors include selecting optimal clinicians, providing them with quality training workshops coupled with ongoing supportive mentoring and consultation, and ongoing program evaluation and monitoring of program fidelity.

It has also become clear to me that successful development and implementation of evidence-based programs requires a serious sustained commitment of personnel and resources. After almost four decades of working at providing research evidence to justify the use of these programs, I can see that bringing about change in parent, teacher, or organizational behaviors requires a committed, persistent, and collaborative team who believe change is possible. Moreover, I have also learned that technology such as video is an important adjunct tool but not sufficient in itself because, in the end, as I learned years ago in Africa, it is the ongoing relationship building that is the key to bringing about innovative change. My mother used to complain that I was always trying to change things. While that is true, I will tell you that I have had fun doing this, and seeing the positive changes in children, and their relationships with their parents and teachers makes it well worth the effort.

Acknowledgement

I wish to thank NIH, NIMH, NINR, and NIDA for 30 years of funding to undertake this research. My NIH *Research Scientist Award* was especially helpful to supporting my personal ability to continue to deliver parent and child groups myself as well as supporting a clinic to deliver both prevention and treatment programs for young children and their parents and teachers.

References

Ainsworth, M. (1974). Infant-mother attachment and social development: Socialization as a product of reciprocal responsiveness to signals. In M. Richards (Ed.), *The integration of the child into the social world*. Cambridge: Cambridge University Press.
Bandura, A. (1977). *Social learning theory*. Englewood Cliffs, NJ: Prentice-Hall, Inc.

Bandura, A. (1982). Self-efficacy mechanisms in human agency. *American Psychologist*, *84*, 191–215.

Baumrind, D. (1971). Current patterns of parental authority. *Psychology Monographs*, *1*, 1–102.

Beck, A.T. (1979). *Cognitive therapy and emotional disorders*. New York: New American Library.

Bowlby, J. (1980). *Attachment and loss: Loss, sadness, and depression*. New York: Basic Books.

Hanf, E. & Kling, J. (1973). *Facilitating parent-child interactions: A two-stage training model*. Eugene, OR: University of Oregon Medical School.

Kogan, K. & Gordon, B.N. (1975). A mother-instruction program: Documenting change in mother-child interactions. *Child Psychiatry and Human Development*.

Menting, A. T. A., Orobio de Castro, B., & Matthys, W. (2013). Effectiveness of the incredible years parent training to modify disruptive and prosocial child behavior: A meta-analytic review. *Clinical Psychology Review*, *33*(8), 901–913.

Patterson, G., Reid, J., & Dishion, T. (1992). *Antisocial boys: A social interactional approach*, vol. 4. Eugene, OR: Castalia Publishing.

Piaget, J., & Inhelder, B. (1962). *The psychology of the child*. New York: Basic Books.

Webster-Stratton, C. (1984). Randomized trial of two parent-training programs for families with conduct-disordered children. *Journal of Consulting and Clinical Psychology*, *52*(4), 666–678.

Webster-Stratton, C. (1994). Advancing videotape parent training: A comparison study. *Journal of Consulting and Clinical Psychology*, *62*(3), 583–593.

Webster-Stratton, C. (2012). *Collaborating with parents to reduce children's behavior problems: A book for therapists using the incredible years programs*. Seattle, WA: Incredible Years Inc.

Webster-Stratton, C., & McCoy, K. P. (2015). Bringing the Incredible Years programs to scale. In K. P. McCoy & A. Dianna (Eds.), *New directions for child and adolescent development. The science and art, of program dissemination: Strategies, successes, and challenges* (Vol. 149, pp. 81–95).

Webster-Stratton, C., Reid, J., & Marsenich, L. (2014). Improving therapist fidelity during evidence-based practice implementation. *Psychiatric Services*, *65*(6), 789–795.

Chapter 6

Development and Implementation of an Evidence-Based Parent Management Training Intervention
GenerationPMTO

Laura A. Rains, Margrét Sigmarsdóttir, and Marion S. Forgatch

GenerationPMTO

> The best was not good enough.
>
> (Patterson, 1982, p. 1)

GenerationPMTO is a suite of evidence-based interventions that empowers parents with skills that alter family dynamics and open doors to healthy social environments. At the core of our clinical practice and ongoing research is the mission set by Gerald R. Patterson to understand the causes of aggression in children in order to apply this knowledge to effective intervention. Patterson and colleagues at the Oregon Social Learning Center (OSLC) began developing our intervention in the 1960s (Patterson, Jones, Whittier, & Wright, 1965). Their strategy involved testing the theory-based intervention through an iterative process of practice and research, a process that continues today. The parenting program model endures more than 50 years later with fidelity and expanding reach across multiple contexts and populations. GenerationPMTO covers the range of preventive intervention through clinical treatment, serving families with children between two and eighteen years old. Parents are treated as the change agents for their children, their families, and themselves. The model teaches effective parenting strategies to prevent and reduce child and adolescent behavior problems and promote healthy development. Based on Coercion Theory and the Social Interaction Learning model (SIL), GenerationPMTO has been tested experimentally (e.g., Dishion, Forgatch, Chamberlain, & Pelham, 2016; Forehand, Lafko, Parent, & Burt, 2014; Forgatch, Patterson, DeGarmo, & Beldavs, 2009; Patterson, Forgatch, & DeGarmo, 2010). It was not until the turn of the 21st century that we learned to implement the program in real-world community contexts. In this chapter, we discuss the model's evolution in terms of content, process, implementation, and fidelity.

Starting Point

Research studies from the 1940s and 50s reported that psychodynamic and child/adolescent-focused treatments, the most popular approaches at the time, were not producing positive outcomes (e.g., Redl & Wineman, 1957). The ineffectiveness of these interventions inspired a zeitgeist among family psychologists to design effective theory-based treatments. About the same time, B.F. Skinner's behavioral perspective was gaining recognition. Trained in psychodynamic psychology, Patterson's early work in residential treatment for youth and juvenile probation led him to focus on child/adolescent behavior problems. Patterson, a young professor, collaborated with a group of likeminded clinicians (i.e., Sidney Bijou, Connie Hanf, and Robert Wahler) to incorporate behavioral tools within interventions that would produce positive outcomes for children and adolescents and their families. This team created the beginnings of modern parent training approaches.

In those golden days of collaboration amongst developmental theorists and emerging model developers, Patterson and OSLC colleagues shared and learned from fellow innovators such as Urie Bronfenbrenner (Ecological Systems Theory) and Albert Bandura (Social Learning Theory) to enrich the foundation of a *behavioral* parent training model. We also integrated therapeutic strategies from clinicians such as Carlos Sluzki (Strategic Family Therapy) and Salvador Minuchin (Structural Family Therapy), contributing to an intervention that is tailored contextually and delivered sensitively. In subsequent decades, a number of parent training interventions based on this early work have been developed, e.g., Parent-Child Interaction Therapy (PCIT; Eyberg & Robinson, 1982); Incredible Years (Webster-Stratton & Hammond, 1997); TripleP (Sanders, 1999); Family Check-up (Dishion et al., 2008). These programs share several core behavioral components with today's evidence-based parenting programs.

Strategy and Theory of Change

The SIL model specifies that behavior is shaped and maintained through reinforcing contingencies that take place during social interaction in the principal social contexts. For children, the family is seen as the most relevant social environment; as children mature, the model specifies that peers become increasingly important as socializing agents (Forgatch et al., 2016; Patterson, 1982; Patterson et al., 2010). The model also specifies that ecological contexts (e.g., trauma, discrimination, dangerous neighborhood, poverty, stress, substance use, mental health) influence social environments (Dishion et al., 2016). For example, harsh and stressful circumstances have been found to be associated with increases in coercive interactions in family and peer relationships. Rather than intervening on the environment, GenerationPMTO empowers parents with effective tools to reduce coercive family interactions, promote positive parenting practices, and thereby prevent and reduce child and adolescent behavior problems. Coercive parenting includes use of aversive behavior, negative reciprocity, escalation, and negative reinforcement. The core positive parenting practices are social learning based: skill encouragement, limit setting, monitoring, problem solving, and positive involvement. Findings from RCTs using random assignment to GenerationPMTO versus control conditions support the theory-based intervention: GenerationPMTO produces significant reduction in child/adolescent behavior problems, reduction in coercive parenting, and increased positive parenting; the improvements in parenting account for the reduction in child/adolescent behavior problems (Forehand et al., 2014; Forgatch et al., 2009; Patterson et al., 2010). With regard to the ecological perspective, improvements in parenting have been shown to mediate improvement in family contexts, such as parental stress and distress, arrests, and socioeconomic factors, including poverty (Patterson et al., 2010).

One of Patterson's edicts was *Make it better*. Another was *Base changes on rigorous research*. The OSLC group of colleagues (see Acknowledgements) followed an iterative process to apply, test, and refine. An early step addressed issues of measurement. Outcome data from interviews and questionnaires provided little understanding of processes that contribute to the outcomes. Influenced by Roger Barker, who observed behavior in the naturalistic environment and theorized that social settings affect behavior, Patterson and John Reid, who joined the group in the 1970s, developed strategies to observe interactions in key settings (e.g., therapy sessions, parent-child interactions, youngsters' peer interactions, classrooms, and playgrounds). The researchers dealt with logistical problems such as location, type of recording device, and finding the least obtrusive location for the observer/camera while maximizing data collection. Direct observation produced a significant perspective change and has become a hallmark of our theoretical, methodological, and intervention research.

The iterative process between practice and research continues today to ensure that the intervention improves and addresses the needs of families. With the collaboration of our expert colleagues around the world, the combination of randomized controlled trials, long term follow-up, structural equation modeling, latent growth modeling, mediational modeling, and other data analytic approaches have enabled us to improve theoretical perspective and the intervention model. Based on clinical experience and direct observation of therapy and family and peer interactions, the behavioral foundation for the intervention has expanded to become the SIL model illustrated in Figure 6.1.

Creating Content

Early Content—Core Components

In its infancy, our evidence-based parenting program began with three core components: positive and negative contingencies and tracking/monitoring. *Skill encouragement* involves a steady process in which parents shape their children's pro-social behavior using contingent positive reinforcement; parents shine the light on behaviors they want to grow. *Limit setting* uses negative contingencies to interrupt, discourage, and prevent problem behaviors. The

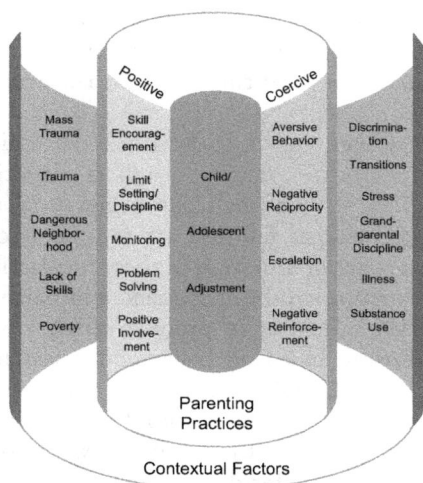

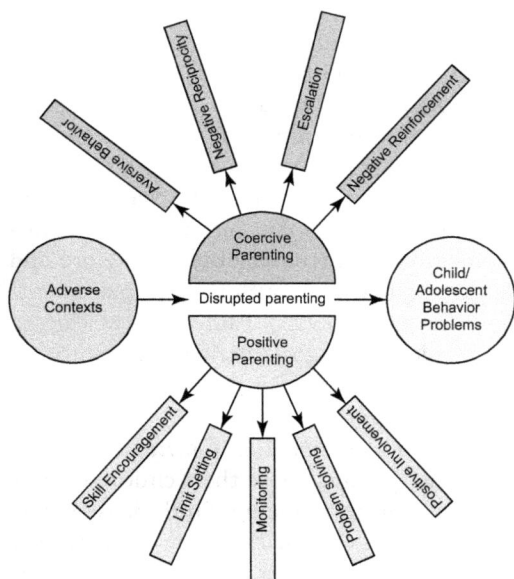

Figure 6.1 A Social Interaction Learning Model

strategies are brief, mild, and delivered in a neutral manner. *Monitoring/supervision/tracking behavior* engages parents' oversight in their children's behavior, activities, whereabouts, and peers to promote safety and healthy surroundings; monitoring is a foundation upon which other parenting skills are constructed (Forgatch, Patterson, & Friend, 2017).

Problem solving was added as a core component to facilitate discussions in which a family can set goals, plan activities, manage conflicts, negotiate agreements, and resolve differences. This story of inclusion began as an offshoot of a standard OSLC assessment that has families attempt to resolve current "hot conflicts." Forgatch was a coder of hundreds of these interactions using an observational system that scored microsocial sequences of behavior among participants. Concerned that the outcomes of problem solving were not rated, she developed a macro measure based on behavioral research of interpersonal problem solving (e.g., Nezu & D'Zurilla, 1981). After scoring the microsocial dimensions, she coded global ratings of problem definition, quality of solutions, extent of resolution, and likelihood of follow through. The items are then formed into a scale score. Her dissertation study found that coercive micro sequences were associated with effective outcomes; problem solving outcomes, in turn, were associated with positive child/youth outcomes (Forgatch, 1989). In another study of interactions between mothers and their confidants, positive problem-solving outcomes were associated with more effective parenting practices (Forgatch & DeGarmo, 1997). Forgatch suggested adding problem solving as a core component to the intervention, but Patterson was unconvinced. He saw problem solving as a cognitive variable and provided a "show me" challenge: Demonstrate that it makes a significant contribution to the model. Forgatch did just that. In a clinical study, improvement in problem-solving outcomes observed before and after treatment predicted a reduction in two-year out-of-home placements and fewer police arrests (Patterson & Forgatch, 1995). Families now learn to use problem-solving strategies (e.g., identify a goal, brainstorm solutions, consider solutions, make a plan, write it down, try it out) in family meetings to provide children with a voice in family matters.

The fifth core component specified in the model is *positive involvement*, which represents the countless ways that parents show their children interest, attention, caring, and love. Rather than introducing child-focused time early on, as is often the practice in some programs with young children, the GenerationPMTO intervention weaves these strategies throughout the intervention. Home practice assignments include spending one-on-one time for conversation, playing games, putting photos in an album, or paying attention to a child's interest. Child-centered activities build family memories and solid relationships. Observations of parent-child interactions before and after intervention have shown improvement in positive involvement (Forgatch & DeGarmo, 2002). Items include parents showing warmth, empathy, affection, and respect toward their children.

Addition of Supporting Components

Over the years we specifically identified a number of supporting components that play a key role in the intervention and, like core components, serve as stand-alone sessions, or are integrated throughout the intervention.

The first supporting component is *good directions*, a strategy that clarifies parents' expectations for children. The intervention has always included a form of *good directions*, but the approach was vague. We developed a specific recipe for parents: Make contact with the child, speak in a firm but friendly manner, say what to do (not what not to do), and then stand and hold until the child gets started. This approach seems easy, but parents can find it hard to put into consistent practice, so we give them a recipe card: [*Name*], *do* [*behavior*] *now, please*. We also practice the recipe using multiple role plays until parents get the strategy under their skin. *Good directions* is often introduced by Session 2 to promote cooperation and prevent noncompliance. Parents learn to follow up their directions with encouragement for cooperation. With a rich supply of skill encouragement comes the introduction of limit setting; noncompliance receives a small negative consequence (e.g., 5- to 10-minute Time Out). Parents from all contexts and cultures tell us that our recipe for clear directions yields increased compliance and inspires a spirit of cooperation in the family (Forgatch & Domenech Rodríguez, 2016).

Another supporting component, *emotions*, emerged to help parents differentiate their own emotions from those of their children and to respond rather than react to situations by regulating their emotions. In the 1980s, Forgatch worked with John Gottman to learn the code for Specific Affects (SPAFF; Gottman, 1988), which is a tool to micro-code the emotional dimension of communication. SPAFF was added as a component of the observational assessment in studies at OSLC. Negative emotions are central aspects of coercive processes in families. A hostile or aversive behavior thrown into the stream of interaction frequently elicits an in-kind response that can escalate, leading to high intensity conflict. For intervention purposes, we engaged a graphic artist to develop materials (e.g., pictures illustrating nonverbal expressions) and created role-play scenarios that illustrate expressions of fear, sadness, anger, contempt, happiness, and interest. Forgatch developed intervention sessions to identify and regulate emotions and first incorporated them in two studies: Oregon Divorce Study (Forgatch, 1994) and Marriage And Parenting in Stepfamilies (MAPS; Forgatch & Rains, 1997). The evolution of this supporting component now includes sessions on identifying and regulating emotions and a gradual integration of the component throughout the intervention. Strategies include up-regulating and down-regulating emotions, especially accompanying *good directions*, encouragement systems, limit setting, family problem solving, and monitoring. All of the populations with whom we work include a substantial portion of families who have experienced trauma. A recent tailoring of the *emotions* component is related specifically to trauma-informed

delivery. Gewirtz and her colleagues adapted GenerationPMTO for returning U.S. military personnel affected by deployment to our wars in Iraq and
Afghanistan. They added mindfulness and emotion coaching components
to the intervention, which were associated with improvements in parenting
and child outcomes, as expected. A new outcome included a reduction in suicide ideation (Gewirtz, DeGarmo, & Zamir, 2016). In another context, in
which we trained child welfare agencies in the GenerationPMTO model, we
added components to increase recognition of signs and symptoms of trauma,
designed practice scenarios to help with emotional experiences in family
reunification, and redoubled our own strengths-based approach throughout
the system that includes parents, practitioners, and child welfare agency staff
(Rains & Forgatch, 2013).

Promoting school success is another supporting component that has its origins
deep in GenerationPMTO history. In the early 1960s, our work focused on
preschool children and their families. As our model incorporated a broader
range of ages and contexts, children's school success became relevant. Research
showed that about half the children with behavior problems at home have
problems at school (Ramsey, Patterson, & Walker, 1990). For these families,
we added strategies to promote academic routines at home emphasizing skill
encouragement bolstered with monitoring children's progress at school. The
skill encouragement element supports children's school-related routines with
token systems, incentive charts, and checklists. The monitoring component
involves activating effective communication between parents and teachers.
The home-school link is strengthened using various techniques that keep parents up to date on their children's homework, school activities, and classroom
behavior. Communication strategies include classroom links, parent-teacher
texting, phone calls, and in-person meetings. In intervention sessions, parents practice active communication, problem solving, and emotion regulation
skills through role play. A goal is to set children up for success for their school
days with academic routines at home. Positive outcomes include improved
quality of homework, reading achievement, and teachers' ratings of children's
adaptive functioning (Forgatch & DeGarmo, 2002).

Active communication is an important supporting component that enhances
united parenting, enables families to navigate the ins and outs of interpersonal problem solving, and helps parents monitor children's activities. The
initial work on communication began with studies in the 1970s as Patterson
and his group applied social learning hypotheses to marital conflict issues
(Patterson, Hops, & Weiss, 1975). We transplanted lessons learned from
couples work to the parent-child and family domain. To make this transfer,
we developed approaches to address parent-child, parent-parent, and family
scenarios. Strategies include making clear goal statements, paying attention
to what and how something is said, taking turns in conversation, observing the perspectives of others, and showing genuine interest and respect. In

the interest of better understanding their children's issues, a communication skillset provides parents with practice simply listening to their children without reacting or giving advice. To promote relationship repair in families whose children have been removed and the goal is reunification, communication activities are integrated with emotional regulation practice (e.g., families create a feelings-themed collage). *Active communication* is introduced in its own session or woven through problem solving, monitoring, and relationship enhancement sessions.

An example of the sequence of GenerationPMTO sessions follows: (1) initial session identifying strengths, setting goals, and noting relevant contextual issues; (2) encouraging cooperation through clear directions; (3) promoting skill development with contingent encouragement; (4) identifying and regulating emotions; (5) setting limits with effective, mild discipline strategies; (6) monitoring children's activities at home and away; (7) communication and interpersonal problem solving; (8) managing conflict within and outside of the family and strengthening the parenting team; (9) promoting school success; and (10) balancing work, love, and play.

Delivering Content

Lessons learned from RCTs and implementing the program with families from differing contexts and cultures led to efforts to improve outcomes. Changes have involved adjusting our approach to intervention. Approximately 30% of our treated clinical cases failed to show significant improvement. To understand the dynamics in such cases, Patterson and Forgatch viewed video recordings of sessions and designed a coding system describing therapist behavior and client responses (Chamberlain et al., 1986). Data revealed that the therapist behaviors of confront and teach elicited "resistance," which was defined as the client's failure to follow the direction set by the therapist. To test the "causal" relationship between the therapists' and clients' behaviors, they conducted an experimental test, manipulating rates of confront and teach within sessions and observing rates of resistance (Patterson & Forgatch, 1985). They found that the combination of confront and teach produced a seven-fold increase in the likelihood that the client's next response would be resistant. An example of confront and teach would be: *No, not like that* (confront). *Let me show you the right way to do it* (teach). The kinds of behaviors labeled resistant were classified as *I can't, I won't, I didn't*, and *family conflict*. Findings from that study led to changes in the process of intervention such that GenerationPMTO therapists learn to teach with support and to avoid confront and teach.

Ensuing "resistance" studies (e.g., Patterson & Chamberlain, 1988; Stoolmiller, Duncan, Bank, & Patterson, 1993) led to an emphasis on the *process* in which *content* is taught by integrating sophisticated clinical skills and active teaching strategies. A host of process skills promotes understanding of content: humor, drama, movement, demonstration, perspective taking, and questioning. The GenerationPMTO teaching approach is "show rather than tell." Therapists model a problem-solving approach that empowers parents, builds rapport, and supports parents as they identify their parenting, family, and children's strengths.

New content and strategies for adapting to specific contexts (e.g., homeless families or those living in supportive housing, military families with a parent at war) continue to be incorporated into the model. Change is based on data, and adaptations are tested with randomized controlled trials. There is more to come about these changes.

Delivery of the intervention is guided by a set of principles. The principles include following an agenda while being responsive to the family, sophisticated clinical skills, and active teaching strategies. Active teaching minimizes verbal teaching and emphasizes learning through practice. Our role-play strategies were strongly influenced by Salvador Minuchin, who visited Patterson's group in the 1980s and taught us to use drama and humor in the process. Our version of role play now has a special twist, something we call the 3D approach: Demonstrate, Differentiate, and Debrief. This involves using sets of mini wrong-way/right-way examples. The practitioner begins with an exaggerated 'wrong-way' example, which often elicits laughter from the parents. To debrief, we ask parents what we did wrong. We write down the parents' critiques, and they become the experts. Then, we brainstorm with the parents how we might do it better, write that down, and try it out. For example, rather than talking through a description of the *good directions* parenting strategy, we throw a pair of shoes across the floor, pretend we're a tired parent walking in the living room after a busy work day, stumble on the shoes, and shout, "What are those #$%^ shoes doing there?! How many times have I ... When will you ever learn ... Why can't you ...!!". By using a dramatic wrong-way role play demonstration, parents experience what it's like as a child to receive an ineffective direction. There's laughter amidst recognition, as the demonstrations are slightly larger than life and nonjudgmental. Wrong-way role plays are debriefed before right-way role plays are used to differentiate the experience and lead parents to insight. Differentiating wrong-way/right-way examples engages parents in the teaching process as collaborators and co-creators. After practitioners model, they have the parents practice, setting the stage for success with specific directions. As the parents role play, practitioners support them with coaching as needed (e.g., whisper coaching, facial expressions, and gestures). Role play debriefings focus on strengths and elicit insights; when needed, we reteach through modeling. Thus, a focus on clinical process skills and active teaching that grew out of the resistance studies impacted our approach to teaching (Forgatch & Domenech Rodríguez, 2016).

Tailoring

As we adapt the intervention for culture and context, we keep a sharp eye on maintaining model adherence. For example, we learned about the best placement of family problem solving during treatment. At the start of our MAPS project, we placed communication and problem solving for couples early in treatment to ensure that newly partnered parents would be able to provide a united parenting front. While it helped to get parents on the same page, they were united in telling us that they wanted to address child behavior issues first. Thus, we changed the order of sessions and started with child behavior, placing the problem solving and communication components later. We offered extra help with these strategies as an early alternative only when the couple needed help with teamwork (Forgatch & DeGarmo, 1997; Forgatch & Rains, 1997). As we address new contexts, we shape the intervention, again with attention to maintaining model fidelity. For example, in the child welfare context where children have been placed in care outside the home and the goal is family reunification, we incorporated modeling/practice scenarios for problem-solving interactions that involve communication with caseworkers, court, and kinship/foster care providers (Forgatch & Rains, 2012).

While Forgatch was collaborating with John Gottman prior to the MAPS study of stepfamilies, we piloted Gottman's oral history interview to include in our assessment battery. Blending families is complicated because they bring with them different histories; by the time couples come to therapy, some of the beauty of forming a new relationship has eroded. The oral history enables couples to see how their family histories differ. It also asks them to describe how they met, what attracted them to one another, and how they became a family, which helps rekindle their early love. This interview produced rapport between assessor and couple and transported the couple back to a time of strengths, a theme that runs throughout GenerationPMTO. The interview created a shared story and understanding: a mini-subculture between the assessor and couple. We had an "Ah-ha" moment when we realized that this journey back to newfound love would promote therapeutic alliance during the intervention's initial session. Thus, we removed the oral history interview from assessment and integrated key elements within our intervention's initial session for stepfamilies; we include it with all two-parent families.

A group of our colleagues began a multi-step process of cultural adaptation to Latinx families that involved an initial adaptation of content and language (Domenech Rodríguez, Baumann, & Schwartz, 2011), followed by trials in Mexico (Amador Buenabad et al., 2019) and Michigan (Parra-Cardona et al., 2017). Rubén Parra-Cardona's work in particular helped inform deep adaptation to the intervention for Latinx parents who were experiencing severe contextual challenges such as chronic poverty, community violence, and immigration-related anxiety (Parra-Cardona, 2019). Melanie Domenech Rodriguez, Parra-Cardona and other bicultural, bilingual colleagues have adapted the

GenerationPMTO intervention to include cultural themes associated with being immigrants and learning to become bicultural families (Parra-Cardona et al., 2012; 2019). Qualitative data indicated protective effects of strengthening parenting skills. Parents described in detail ways in which benefits of the intervention (e.g., child compliance, improved parent-child relationship) created a cognitive buffer to adversity. As parents became more effective and their children's behavior improved, families became more resilient and hope for the future grew. Parents came to understand that although they may not be able to change their larger contexts, they can shape their children's development and emotional wellbeing with nurturing, consistent, and effective parenting practices (Parra-Cardona, 2019).

GenerationPMTO can be delivered in a variety of formats, depending on the population, context, culture, and other factors. Individual delivery employs a principle-based approach with flexible responsiveness to specific family contexts; group facilitators must respond to group dynamics as they maintain a more scripted, agenda-driven weekly format. Within our group of mentors, we have debated whether it is best to train practitioners first in group delivery, with its clear and somewhat rigid structure, and then follow up with individual delivery training, or *vice versa*. Individual delivery allows a deeper understanding of the principles underlying the intervention. The group format enables practitioners to move through the program without getting stuck on a single component, thus lengthening treatment or disengagement before completion. The Michigan PMTO implementation site is training with both options and may yield an answer to our question.

Refining, Expanding, Implementing

In this section, we describe the evolution of our implementation model, which includes training, coaching, fidelity, and sustainability. We also discuss the expansion of GenerationPMTO into communities and systems of care in the U.S. and internationally. Finally, we describe our more recent foray into the world of marketing to increase access to our program for families who need it most.

Even though we arrived late to implementation relative to some other parenting programs, the roots of GenerationPMTO in the parent training community are deep and wide. The work of Patterson and colleagues provided a strong foundation from which Forgatch and her team could respond to requests to implement GenerationPMTO in systems of care. One option would have been to blaze into a community without taking into account contextual factors relevant for the local population and apply the parenting program with a one-size-fits-all approach. Why not just hand parents a principle-based book, wish them well, and hope for the best? Besides the disrespect, it is a set up for failure. Consider what would happen if someone gave you a direction that may be clear to them but has no relevance to your language, culture, context, and lived experience. Message sent does not necessarily equal message received.

We were fortunate that our first full-scale project provided us with support as we learned how to implement. At the request of the Norwegian Ministries of Health and Child & Family Welfare, we traveled to Norway in the late 1990s to train a cohort of 40 practitioners (Askeland, Forgatch, Apeland, Reer, & Grønlie, 2019; Forgatch & DeGarmo, 2011). This implementation project required developing training strategies that could be carried out nationwide, in another culture, nearly 5,000 miles away across the North Pole. We were living in the era of overhead projectors, plastic transparencies, and bulky laptops, all of which made for a heavy footprint and oversized luggage. We learned to train, guided by Nancy Knutson, a school psychologist with expertise in adult learning methods. Our training team began with Forgatch and Knutson, and soon included Laura Rains, a clinical social worker. Rains is now the Director of Implementation and Training for GenerationPMTO. She adapts implementation designs for specific sites and leads the training of practitioners, trainers, and coaches. Margrét Sigmarsdóttir joined in 2007 and has since become the leader of the GenerationPMTO Fidelity of Implementation (FIMP) Consensus team, which monitors international fidelity teams.

Training Therapists

GenerationPMTO training uses best-practice adult-learning methods supplemented with detailed practitioner manuals and materials, parent materials, and a reading list of book chapters and journal articles to promote model understanding at a deep level. The training program is active, structured, and responsive to context. We demonstrate ineffective and effective therapeutic approaches to help trainees develop insight into strategies that prevent and reduce parents' resistance to the techniques. Workshop seminars take place in a comfortable learning environment with plenty of practice to promote mastery. Immediately after the first workshop, practitioners begin session work in their community agencies. They receive virtual, in-person, and written coaching based on observations of video-recorded therapy sessions. Most communities use our web-based, HIPAA-compliant database system that tracks progress of practitioners' family work, stores fidelity scores, provides space for uploading recorded sessions to enable coaching, and enhances communication. Over the training period, practitioners work with a minimum of five families, two of which function as "certification families" (Sigmarsdóttir, Rains, & Forgatch, 2016).

Training includes in-person workshops and coaching based on video recordings of intervention sessions. This observation-based coaching is provided with written feedback and group or individual coaching in-person or virtually. Trainees learn how to implement the GenerationPMTO intervention with parents with use of role plays and emphasis on effective process skills. In our earliest days, we provided 18 workshop days and the training process lasted 18 months to two years. This approach has been shown to be successful. For example, in Norway, 24% of the therapists we trained in the first cohort of practitioners beginning in 1999 maintained their practice with certification 17 years later (Askeland et al., 2019). However, other implementation sites tell us that such a timeline is too long for contexts in which demands are high and, frankly, there is competition from other programs with briefer training formats. While some GenerationPMTO sites continue to use the 18-day training format, today, our typical certification program includes a minimum of 10 days of in-person/virtual workshop days with regular observation-based coaching. When practitioners begin family service delivery immediately after the first workshop, certification as a GenerationPMTO Specialist can be achieved as early as eight months, although it typically takes 12 to 18 months.

Coaching

In GenerationPMTO, observation-based coaching supports competent adherence to the model. Coaching is provided for individual practitioners or group leaders, with feedback in written or verbal format or, in most cases, both. In the mid-2000s, we added group reflective coaching to our feedback procedures. Mona Duckert, a Norwegian psychologist and GenerationPMTO colleague, trained us in reflective coaching, which we incorporated in our Michigan and Netherlands implementations. The practice continues to be a staple of coaching at all sites. Key benefits include promoting a safe environment for learning and focusing on strengths while not flooding the practitioner. Feedback is presented through the lens of the program's fidelity system, FIMP (Knutson, Forgatch, Rains, Sigmarsdóttir, & Domenech Rodríguez, 2019). Takeaways from coaching are identified for application in coming sessions. The agenda begins by asking the coachee to describe the family and present a coaching question. Then the group observes a session segment that lasts about 10 minutes, which is followed by discussion between the coach and coachee. The coach later invites input from a reflective team of practitioners and leads practice within the group. Regular coaching is an integral component of GenerationPMTO, both during training and afterwards to help therapists deepen their skills and address difficult issues during family work.

GenerationPMTO is known for being strengths-based with parents and with clinicians. Ironically, it is not uncommon to receive pushback for being *too* positive with feedback. For example, clinicians from one implementation site stated that they were used to receiving criticism, being told only what they were doing wrong clinically: "This took a whole shift in perspective. And now we've learned to read between the lines. But when we first started and [were] getting that feedback, it was like, what is all this rainbows and unicorn stuff?" (Akin, 2016, pp. 162–164). Now we clarify our intentions with practitioners upfront, stating that we will be using a strengths-based coaching approach (e.g., *When we say something went well, we mean do it again*). We follow the model's *5:1 principle*; for every correction, we shine the light on five positives about what is done well. We also take care to provide constructive feedback for further practice.

Fidelity and Sustainability

The GenerationPMTO program highlights fidelity as an essential implementation component and the developers invest considerable resources in FIMP, the observation-based measurement tool. FIMP evaluates model adherence in terms of both content and competent delivery. Studies have evaluated the predictive validity of FIMP (i.e., high fidelity scores predict positive outcomes). The first test of FIMP was an efficacy trial in Oregon with an at-risk prevention sample of stepfamilies; high FIMP scores predicted improvements in observed parenting practices (Forgatch, Patterson, & DeGarmo, 2005). Researchers replicated these findings in a Norwegian implementation study with 110 therapists and 242 families, showing that high FIMP scores predicted pre/post change in parenting practices (Forgatch & DeGarmo, 2011) and pre/post change in child behavior as rated by their parents (Hukkelberg & Ogden, 2013).

Fidelity is monitored in all GenerationPMTO sites on an annual basis to ensure long-term sustainability with high fidelity. In GenerationPMTO's *full transfer approach* to implementation, the program developers train the first generation of practitioners to certification; then they train trainers, coaches, and fidelity raters within the site. Thus, subsequent generations are trained by the adopting community. Two recent European studies indicate that reach can be extended significantly while sustaining high levels of fidelity for decades (Askeland et al., 2019; Sigmarsdóttir et al., 2019).

Expansion

Today GenerationPMTO has been installed in several locations in North America, including in the U.S., Mexico City in Mexico, and the province of British Colombia in Canada. The program has also been implemented nationwide in Norway, Iceland, Denmark, and the Netherlands. GenerationPMTO has been adapted for different ethnic groups within and outside of implementation sites, including Somali and Pakistani immigrant mothers in Norway (Bjørknes, Kjøbli, Manger, & Jakobsen, 2012), Somali parents in Minnesota (Gewirtz, Mohammad, Orieny, & Yaylaci, 2011), Spanish-speaking Latinx families in a rural community in Utah (Domenech Rodríguez et al., 2011), in an urban Latinx community in Detroit, Michigan (Parra-Cardona et al., 2017), war-affected families in Northern Uganda (Wieling et al., 2015), and in a project for military families in Minnesota (Gewirtz, DeGarmo, & Zamir, 2018). Most of those projects have been tested with randomized controlled trials; others have been tested for feasibility.

Dissemination and Marketing

For a long time, the main marketing tool for GenerationPMTO was word of mouth, publications, conferences, and satisfied sites. People came to us through those channels. In the last decade, however, we incorporated professional marketing tools to promote our program and implement more broadly. We hired a marketing firm. They asked us to explain who we are and what we do, which helped us to clarify our vision. Along the way we rebranded from Parent Management Training – Oregon Model (PMTO) to GenerationPMTO, emerged with a professional logo, and found our team's strengths in designing promotional materials, creating monthly newsletters, and posting on social media. We also became more aware of selling our time and materials rather than giving them away.

Lessons Learned

Over the course of 50 years, we have learned a lot from hardworking community members who put research into action with families around the globe. Here are some highlights of what designing and sustaining an evidence-based program has taught us.

- In the words of Patterson: "Always strive to make your intervention better."
- Use active teaching skills to engage parents in the learning process. Our approach uses problem solving and extensive role play for rehearsal, which parents find fun and empowering.
- To reduce parental resistance, avoid combining confrontation with teaching (e.g., *not that way, this way*). Instead, join and provide a supportive context for brainstorming (e.g., *yes, that is difficult, let's consider some ideas*).
- Coach and train using video recordings of session material to fine-tune practitioner skills, address resistance, and troubleshoot problems.
- Monitor fidelity and intervention outcomes; adjust components, theoretical perspective, and assessment as necessary. For example, review "failed" cases to identify ways to improve.
- Provide intervention in relevant languages and collaborate with local sites to adapt and use culturally appropriate metaphors and concepts.
- Adopt before adapt. Maintain core intervention components as tailor to address relevant contextual and cultural circumstances.
- Base changes in the program's theoretical and intervention models on data.
- Engage players at all levels (e.g., front-line clinical, assessment and intake staff, clinical supervisors and directors, leadership and champions) to preempt problems and troubleshoot solutions.
- Create opportunities for onsite visits and meetings across regional lines.

Closing

We have described the evolution of GenerationPMTO content and process and our efforts to extend our reach with large-scale implementations. When we are invited in—whether by family or community—we join, focus on strengths, exchange information, determine goals, emphasize commonalities, and tailor applications through a collaborative process. The art and science of this process is essential at all levels of practice. Like many leading programs, our group is forever striving to improve, respond to change, grow with fidelity, and follow Patterson's call to *make it better* and *base change on data*. Inspired by Patterson and the group that he formed in the 1960s and 70s, we continue to address those calls to make the world a better place, especially for families most in need of effective intervention.

Acknowledgments

The authors wish to acknowledge early contributors to the theory and practice underpinning the GenerationPMTO model, including, in alphabetical order: Patricia Chamberlain, Tom Dishion, Beverly Fagot, Marion Forgatch, Jerry Patterson, and John Reid. Methodological innovations by Lew Bank, Dave DeGarmo, and Mike Stoolmiller placed our group at OSLC on the cutting edge. Our own growth in implementation would not have occurred without guidance from Nancy Knutson and our initial collaboration with Norwegian colleagues across the North Pole, each implementation leader since, and invaluable staff past and present at ISII and OSLC. Most importantly, the development and application of this model is due to the dedicated parents and practitioners who take the extra steps to make positive family change a reality.

We are indebted to Kelly Bryson for her thorough and cheerful editorial support.

Funding Information

We acknowledge support that funded much of the work: Grant No. R01 MH 38318 from the Child and Adolescent Treatment and Preventive Intervention Research Branch, DSIR, NIMH, U.S. PHS Grant No. RO1DA 16097 from the Prevention Research Branch, NIDA, US PHS, Forgatch PI; Grant No. R01 MH 54703 from the Child and Adolescent Treatment and Preventive Intervention Research Branch, DSIR, NIMH, U.S. PHS, Forgatch PI; Grant No. R01 DA 16097 from the Prevention Research Branch, NIDA, U.S. PHS, Forgatch PI; Grant No. P30 MH 46690 Prevention and Behavioral Medicine Research Branch, Division of Epidemiology and Services Research, NIMH & ORMH, U.S. PHS, Reid PI; Grant No. R37 MH 37940 from the Antisocial and Other Personality Disorders Program, NIMH, U.S. PHS, Patterson PI through 1998, then Capaldi PI; Grant No. W81XWH-16-1-0407 from the United States Department of Defense, Gewirtz PI; and Grant No. 1U79SM080009-01 from the U.S. Department of Health and Human Services, SAMHSA, Gewirtz PI.

References

Akin, B. A. (2016). Practitioner views on the core functions of coaching in the implementation of an evidence-based intervention in child welfare. *Children and Youth Services Review, 68,* 159–168. doi: 10.1016/j.childyouth.2016.07.010

Amador Buenabad, N. G., Sánchez Ramos, R., Díaz Juárez, A. D., Gutiérrez López, M. d. L., Ortiz Gallegos, A. B., González Ortega, T. G., ... Villatoro Velázquez, J. A. (2019). Cluster randomized trial of a multicomponent school-based program in Mexico to prevent behavioral problems and develop social skills in children. *Frontiers,* Online first 3 December. doi: 10.1007/s10566-019-09535-3

Askeland, E., Forgatch, M., Apeland, A., Reer, M., & Grønlie, A. A. (2019). Scaling up an empirically supported intervention with long-term outcomes: The nationwide implementation of GenerationPMTO in Norway. *Prevention Science,* Online first 23 August. doi: 10.1007/s11121-019-01047-9

Bjørknes, R., Kjøbli, J., Manger, T., & Jakobsen, R. (2012). Parent training among ethnic minorities: Parenting practices as mediators of change in child conduct problems. *Family Relations: An Interdisciplinary Journal of Applied Family Studies, 61*(1), 101–114. doi: 10.1111/j.1741-3729.2011.00683.x

Chamberlain, P., Davis, B., Forgatch, M. S., Frey, S., Patterson, G. R., Ray, J. R., ... Trombley, T. (1986). *The therapy process code: An observational system. Inhouse manuscript/code.* Eugene, OR: Oregon Social Learning Center.

Dishion, T. J., Connell, A., Weaver, C., Shaw, D., Gardner, F., & Wilson, M. (2008). The Family Check-Up with high-risk indigent families: Preventing problem behavior by increasing parents' positive behavior support in early childhood. *Child Development, 79*(5), 1395–1414. doi: 10.1111/j.1467-8624.2008.01195.x

Dishion, T. J., Forgatch, M. S., Chamberlain, P., & Pelham, W. E. (2016). The Oregon model of behavior family therapy: From intervention design to promoting large-scale system change. *Behavior Therapy (Special Issue), 47*(6), 812–837. doi: 10.1016/j.beth.2016.02.002

Domenech Rodríguez, M. M., Baumann, A. A., & Schwartz, A. L. (2011). Cultural adaptation of an evidence based intervention: From theory to practice in a Latino/a community context. *American Journal of Community Psychology, 47*(1–2), 170–186. doi: 10.1007/s10464-010-9371-4

Eyberg, S. M., & Robinson, E. A. (1982). Parent-child interaction training: Effects on family functioning. *Journal of Clinical Child Psychology, 11,* 130–137. doi: 10.1080/15374418209533076

Forehand, R., Lafko, N., Parent, J., & Burt, K. B. (2014). Is parenting the mediator of change in behavioral parent training for externalizing problems of youth? *Clinical Psychology Review, 34*(8), 608–619. doi: 10.1016/j.cpr.2014.10.001

Forgatch, M. S. (1989). Patterns and outcome in family problem solving: The disrupting effect of negative emotion. *Journal of Marriage and Family, 51*(1), 115–124. doi: 10.2307/352373

Forgatch, M. S. (1994). *Parenting through change: A programmed intervention curriculum for groups of single mothers.* [Unpublished training manual]. Eugene, OR: Oregon Social Learning Center.

Forgatch, M. S., & DeGarmo, D. S. (1997). Adult problem solving: Contributor to parenting and child outcomes in divorced families. *Social Development*, 6(2), 238–254. doi: 10.1111/j.1467-9507.1997.tb00104.x

Forgatch, M. S., & DeGarmo, D. S. (2002). Extending and testing the social interaction learning model with divorce samples. In J. B. Reid, G. R. Patterson & J. Snyder (Eds.), *Antisocial behavior in children and adolescents: A developmental analysis and model for intervention* (pp. 235–256). Washington, DC: American Psychological Association.

Forgatch, M. S., & DeGarmo, D. S. (2011). Sustaining fidelity following the nationwide PMTO implementation in Norway. *Prevention Science*, 12(3), 235–246. doi: 10.1007/s11121-011-0225-6

Forgatch, M. S., & Domenech Rodríguez, M. M. (2016). Interrupting coercion: The iterative loops among theory, science, and practice. In T. J. Dishion & Snyder, J. J. (Eds.), *The Oxford handbook of coercive relationship dynamics* (pp. 194–214). New York: Oxford University Press.

Forgatch, M. S., Patterson, G. R., & DeGarmo, D. S. (2005). Evaluating fidelity: Predictive validity for a measure of competent adherence to the Oregon model of parent management training (PMTO). *Behavior Therapy*, 36(1), 3–13. doi: 10.1016/S0005-7894(05)80049-8

Forgatch, M. S., Patterson, G. R., DeGarmo, D. S., & Beldavs, Z. G. (2009). Testing the Oregon delinquency model with 9-year follow-up of the Oregon Divorce Study. *Development and Psychopathology*, 21(2), 637–660. doi: 10.1017/S0954579409000340

Forgatch, M. S., Patterson, G. R., & Friend, T. (2017). *Raising cooperative kids: Proven practices for a connected, happy family*. Newburyport, MA: Conari Press.

Forgatch, M. S., & Rains, L. A. (1997). *MAPS: marriage and parenting in stepfamilies*. [Unpublished training manual]. Eugene, OR: Oregon Social Learning Center.

Forgatch, M. S., & Rains, L. A. (2012). *Parenting through change – Preparing for reunification CSNYC*. [Unpublished training manual]. Eugene, OR: Implementation Sciences International, Inc.

Forgatch, M. S., Snyder, J. J., Patterson, G. R., Pauldine, M. R., Chaw, Y., Elish, K., … Richardson, E. B. (2016). Resurrecting the Chimera: Progressions in parenting and peer processes. *Development and Psychopathology (Special Issue)*, 28(3), 689–706. doi: 10.1017/S0954579416000250

Gewirtz, A. H., DeGarmo, D. S., & Zamir, O. (2016). Effects of military parenting program on parental distress and suicidal ideation: After deployment adaptive parenting tools. *Suicide and Life Threatening Behaviors*, 46(Suppl.1), S23–S31. doi: 10.1111/sltb.12255

Gewirtz, A. H., DeGarmo, D. S., & Zamir, O. (2018). After deployment, adaptive parenting tools: One year outcomes of an evidence-based parenting program for military families. *Prevention Science*, 19(4), 589–599. doi: 10.1007/s11121-017-0839-4

Gewirtz, A. H., Mohammad, J., Orieny, P., & Yaylaci, F. T. (2011). Adapting trauma interventions for refugee families. *The Dialogue*, 7(2), 2–3. Rockville, MD: SAMHSA.

Gottman, J. M. (1988). *Observing emotional communication in marital and family interaction: SPAFF manual*. [Unpublished training manual] University of Washington Department of Psychology, Seattle, WA.

Hukkelberg, S., & Ogden, T. (2013). Working alliance and treatment fidelity as predictors of externalizing problem behaviors in Parent Management Training. *Journal of Consulting and Clinical Psychology*, 81(6), 1010–1020. doi: 10.1037/a0033825

Knutson, N. M., Forgatch, M. S., Rains, L. A., Sigmarsdóttir, M., & Domenech Rodríguez, M. M. (2019). *Fidelity of Implementation Rating System (FIMP): The manual for GenerationPMTO* (3rd ed.). [Unpublished training manual]. Eugene, OR: Implementation Sciences International, Inc.

Nezu, A. M., & D'Zurilla, T. J. (1981). Effects of problem definition and formulation on the generation of alternatives in the social problem-solving process. *Cognitive Theory and Research*, *5*(3), 265–271. doi: 10.1007/BF01193410

Parra-Cardona, J. R. (2019). Healing through parenting: An intervention delivery and process of change model developed with low-income Latina/o (Latinx) immigrant families. *Family Process*, *58*(1), 34–52. doi: 10.1111/famp.12429

Parra-Cardona, J. R., Bybee, D., Sullivan, C. M., Domenech Rodríguez, M. M., Dates, B., Tams, L., & Bernal, G. (2017). Examining the impact of differential cultural adaptation with Latina/o immigrants exposed to adapted parent training interventions. *Journal of Consulting and Clinical Psychology*, *85*(1), 58–71. doi: 10.1037/ccp0000160

Parra-Cardona, J. R., Domenech Rodríguez, M. M., Forgatch, M. S., Sullivan, C., Bybee, D., Holtrop, K., ... Bernal, G. (2012). Culturally adapting an evidence-based parenting intervention for Latino immigrants: The Need to integrate fidelity and cultural relevance. *Family Process*, *51*(1), 56–72. doi: 10.1111/j.1545-5300.2012.01386.x

Parra-Cardona, R., López-Zerón, G., Leija, S. G., Maas, M. K., Villa, M., Zamudio, E., ... Domenech Rodríguez, M. M. (2019). A culturally adapted intervention for Mexican-origin parents of adolescents: The need to overtly address culture and discrimination in evidence-based practice. *Family Process*, *58*(2), 334–352. doi: 10.1111/famp.12381

Patterson, G. R. (1982). *A social learning approach: Coercive family process*. Eugene, OR: Castalia.

Patterson, G. R., & Chamberlain, P. (1988). Treatment process: A problem at three levels. In L. C. Wynne (Ed.), *The state of the art in family therapy research: Controversies and recommendations* (pp. 189–223). New York: Family Process Press.

Patterson, G. R., & Forgatch, M. S. (1985). Therapist behavior as a determinant for client noncompliance: A paradox for the behavior modifier. *Journal of Consulting and Clinical Psychology*, *53*(6), 846–851. doi: 10.1037/0022-006X.53.6.846

Patterson, G. R., & Forgatch, M. S. (1995). Predicting future clinical adjustment from treatment outcome and process variables. *Psychological Assessment*, *7*(3), 275–285. doi: 10.1037/1040-3590.7.3.275

Patterson, G. R., Forgatch, M. S., & DeGarmo, D. S. (2010). Cascading effects following intervention. *Development and Psychopathology*, *22*(4), 949–970. doi: 10.1017/S0954579410000568

Patterson, G. R., Hops, H., & Weiss, R. L. (1975). Interpersonal skill training for couples in early stages of conflict. *Journal of Marriage and Family*, *37*(2), 295–303. doi: 10.2307/350963

Patterson, G. R., Jones, R. R., Whittier, J., & Wright, M. A. (1965). A behavior modification technique for the hyperactive child. *Behavior Research and Therapy*, *2*(2–4), 217–226. doi: 10.1016/0005-7967(64)90019-1

Rains, L. A., & Forgatch, M. S. (2013). Trauma-informed PMTO: An adaptation of the Oregon Model of Parent Management Training. *Trauma-Informed Child Welfare Practice*, Winter, *24*, 38–42.

Ramsey, E., Patterson, G. R., & Walker, H. M. (1990). Generalization of the antisocial trait from home to school settings. *Journal of Applied Developmental Psychology*, *11*(2), 209–223. doi: 10.1016/0193-3973(90)90006-6

Redl, F., & Wineman, D. (1957). *The aggressive child*. New York: The Free Press.

Sanders, M. R. (1999). Triple P-Positive Parenting Program: Towards an empirically validated multilevel parenting and family support strategy for the prevention of behavior and emotional problems in children. *Clinical Child and Family Psychology Review*, *2*(2), 71–90. doi: 10.1023/A:1021843613840

Sigmarsdóttir, M., Forgatch, M. S., Guðmundsdóttir, E. V., Thorlacius, Ö., Svendsen, G. T., Tjaden, J., & Gewirtz, A. H. (2019). Implementing an evidence-based intervention for children in Europe: Evaluating the full-transfer approach. *Journal of Clinical Child and Adolescent Psychology*, *48*(Suppl.1), S312–S325. doi: 10.1080/15374416.2018.1466305

Sigmarsdóttir, M., Rains, L. A., & Forgatch, M. S. (2016). Parent Management Training - Oregon Model (PMTO): A program to treat children's behavior problems. In J. J. Ponzetti (Ed.), *Evidence-based parenting education: A global perspective* (pp. 192–205). New York: Taylor & Francis/Psychology Press.

Stoolmiller, M., Duncan, T. E., Bank, L., & Patterson, G. R. (1993). Some problems and solutions in the study of change: Significant patterns of client resistance. *Journal of Consulting and Clinical Psychology*, *61*(6), 920–928. doi: 10.1037/0022-006X.61.6.920

Webster-Stratton, C., & Hammond, M. (1997). Treating children with early-onset conduct problems: A comparison of child and parent training interventions. *Journal of Consulting and Clinical Psychology*, *65*(1), 93–109. doi: 10.1037/0022-006X.65.1.93

Wieling, E., Mehus, C., Mollerherm, J., Neuner, F., Laura, A., & Catani, C. (2015). Assessing the feasibility of providing a parenting intervention for war affected families in Northern Uganda. *Family and Community Health*, *38*(3), 252–267. doi: 10.1097/FCH.0000000000000064

Chapter 7

Developing the Triple P System as a Population Approach to Parenting Support

Matthew R. Sanders

The Starting Point

The Triple P-Positive Parenting Program (hereafter referred to as the "Triple P system") is a unique, population based, multilevel system of evidence-based parenting support targeting children from infancy through to adolescence (Sanders & Mazzucchelli, 2018). The beginnings of Triple P date back to 1978 when I developed a 10-session parenting intervention delivered individually to parents of disruptive preschool-aged children in their homes through active skills training. This was completed as part of my PhD, under the mentorship of my primary doctoral supervisor Professor Ted Glynn (The University of Auckland), advisor Professor Todd Risley (University of Kansas), and supervisor Professor Jack James (the University of Queensland). An article by Sanders and Glynn (1981) comprised the foundation evidence supporting the program's effectiveness.

The intervention focused on using self-management training to help parents generalize their application of positive parenting and contingency management procedures to diverse settings. Parents were initially trained in one setting (home) and a self-management procedure taught parents to adapt strategies to additional home and community settings (e.g., shopping, visiting, bedtime), and to other siblings. This initial intervention eventually became known as Standard Triple P.

In 1979, I joined the academic staff of the University of Queensland (UQ). I completed my doctoral studies in psychology in 1981 and have worked continuously at UQ for four decades at the time of writing, first in the Department of Psychiatry (1979–1995) and then in the School of Psychology, where I established the Parenting and Family Support Centre (PFSC) (1996 to present). This center has been the research and development base for Triple P from 1996 to the present. It is also involved in the training for clinical, child, and family psychologists completing Masters and PhDs at UQ.

Several key individuals inspired my approach to parenting support. Ted Glynn introduced me to the power of applied behavior analysis (ABA) and applications of self-management procedures (self-determination of goals, self-monitoring, self-evaluation, self-reinforcement) in classroom settings (Ballard & Glynn, 1975), which led me to become curious to explore the application of self-management with parents of children with serious behavior problems. Children with conduct problems interested me because of their disruptive influence in classroom setting and adverse effects on teachers, parents, and peers. ABAs focus on the use of objective observational measures of outcome, precision in the depiction of intervention methods based on learning principles (functional analysis, stimulus control, consequences, contingencies). ABAs often take advantage of the value of intra-subject replication designs, and single case methods were particularly appealing. At the time in 1978, the ABA field had only a limited focus on parenting interventions. Todd Risley was renowned for his intervention research on living environments for dependent people (from infants to the elderly). His work was a powerful exemplar of how to integrate specific behavior change procedures to teach new skills and behaviors with careful planning of contextual, organizational, and environmental issues. Albert Bandura's work on cognitive social learning theory (1977) informed our model of parental self-regulation (Sanders, Turner & Metzler, 2019), which led us to target cognitive mechanisms (expectations, beliefs, attributions) and utilize social learning-based strategies (video modeling) in parenting interventions to facilitate parental skill acquisition. Jerry Patterson's seminal work at the Oregon Social Learning Center on coercive family processes with severe conduct problems was a great example of using observational methods to describe and understand parent-child interaction (e.g., coercive escalation) and to evaluate parenting interventions (Patterson, Reid, Jones, & Conger, 1975). Finally, I became interested in public health after visiting the Stanford Heart Disease Prevention Project at Stanford University in 1983 while on sabbatical leave. I was impressed by the integrated use of behavioral sciences including communication theory, social learning theory, and behavior change strategies as part of an integrated public health approach. I became convinced that a whole of population, multi-level approach to parenting support was needed to prevent social, emotional, and behavioral problems, and child maltreatment in children. This was a turning point for me to start thinking about parenting at a population level rather than just in terms of treatments for individual clinical cases and disorders.

From 1978 to 1993 I started researching the effects of positive parenting under a generic name, the Family Intervention Research Project. In these 15 years I developed a team that gradually built a comprehensive five-level system of parenting intervention that exists today, and we named it the Triple P-Positive Parenting Program in 1993.

Strategy and Theory of Change

Triple P evolved to address the limitations of the prevailing individual and group treatment models of parent training for dealing with children's social and emotional problems. Clinic-based parent training approaches only reached a small proportion of children with conduct problems, and most vulnerable and disadvantaged children did not receive any intervention. The multilevel approach we developed aimed to increase the population reach of the intervention and to avoid the "one size fits all" approach to intervention. Flexible modes of delivery were used to ensure that as many families as possible could participate regardless of where they live. The recognition that in a country as vast as Australia, where geographical isolation of parents often meant lack of access to services, it became essential to explore whether use of technology (e.g., use of telephone- based delivery and eventually the internet) could be used to overcome barriers to participation. The main obstacle was lack of opportunity to directly observe parent-child interaction to provide feedback to parents about implementation challenges. Despite this limitation parents benefited greatly from the combination of text materials and telephone consultation, and later from an interactive online format (Day & Sanders, 2018; Morawska & Sanders, 2006). Most Triple P variants can now be accessed via telephone-based support, text-based self-help or online delivery. Triple P's blended model of intervention incorporated both universal and targeted elements, low intensity programs for all parents, and a tiered continuum of increasingly intensive interventions for more complex cases. Not all parents require the same level of professional support. This notion of a tiered, multilevel system is represented in in Figure 7.1. From the early 1990s our team in the PFSC decided that each new program variant, level of intensity, and

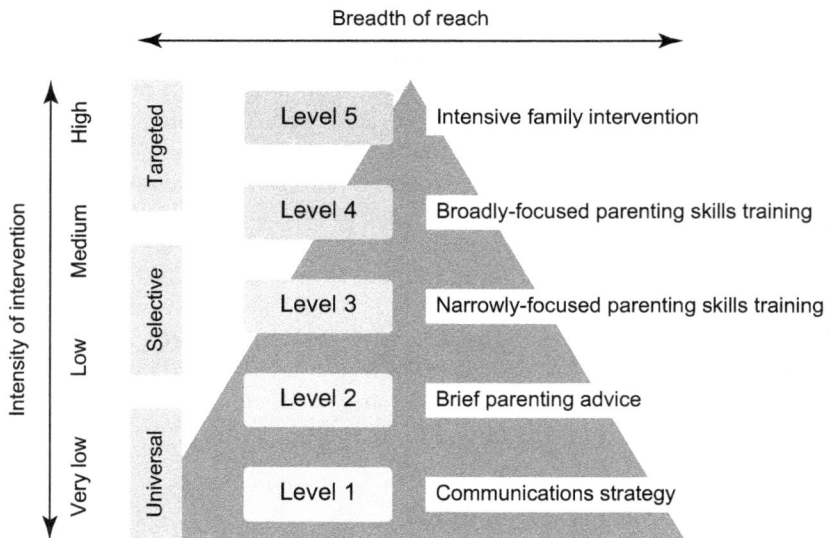

Figure 7.1 The Triple P Multilevel System of Parenting Support

delivery modality needed to have sufficient evidence of effectiveness before the variant became part of the system. The programs include both prevention and treatment interventions and target age groups from pre-birth through to adolescence.

In designing parent resources we aimed to be as procedurally specific as possible in describing individual parenting techniques and their application to different types of child behavior (e.g., tantrums, whining) in various parenting situations (e.g., taking children shopping, bedtime). Seventeen core-parenting skills relevant to parenting of children (0–12 years) became the core parenting skills (see Table 7.1). The specific details of the parenting techniques and principles of effective usage of these skills were derived from learning theory and its application in various applied settings. The decision

Table 7.1 Core Parenting Principles and Skills Promoted in Triple P for Children Aged 0–12 Years

Safe and Engaging Environment	Positive Learning Environment	Assertive Discipline	Realistic Expectations	Parental Self- Care
Spending brief quality time	Giving nonverbal attention	Establishing ground rules	Monitoring children's behavior	Catching unhelpful thoughts
Talking with children	Giving descriptive praise	Using directed discussion	Setting developmentally appropriate goals	Using relaxation and stress management
Showing affection	Setting a good example	Using planned ignoring	Setting practice tasks	Developing personal coping statements
Providing engaging activities	Using incidental teaching	Giving clear, calm instructions	Self-evaluating strengths and weaknesses	Challenging unhelpful thoughts
	Using "ask-say-do"	Using logical consequences	Setting personal goals for change	Developing coping plans for high-risk situations
	Using behavior charts	Using brief interruption		Improving personal communication habits
		Using quiet time		Giving and receiving constructive feedback
		Using time-out		Having casual conversations
				Supporting each other when problem behavior occurs

Table 7.2 Triple P Logic Model for Reducing Child Maltreatment

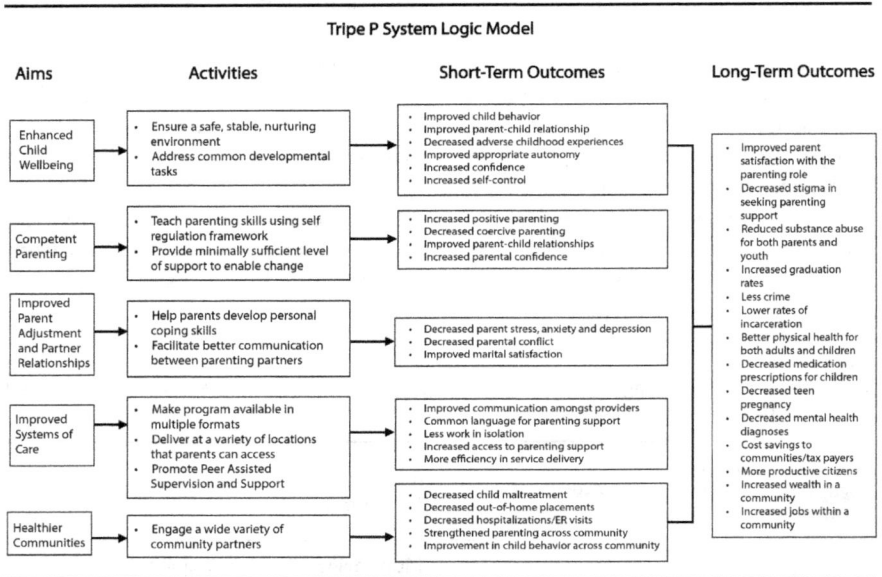

Tripe P System Logic Model

Aims	Activities	Short-Term Outcomes	Long-Term Outcomes
Enhanced Child Wellbeing	• Ensure a safe, stable, nurturing environment • Address common developmental tasks	• Improved child behavior • Improved parent-child relationship • Decreased adverse childhood experiences • Improved appropriate autonomy • Increased confidence • Increased self-control	• Improved parent satisfaction with the parenting role • Decreased stigma in seeking parenting support • Reduced substance abuse for both parents and youth • Increased graduation rates • Less crime • Lower rates of incarceration • Better physical health for both adults and children • Decreased medication prescriptions for children • Decreased teen pregnancy • Decreased mental health diagnoses • Cost savings to communities/tax payers • More productive citizens • Increased wealth in a community • Increased jobs within a community
Competent Parenting	• Teach parenting skills using self regulation framework • Provide minimally sufficient level of support to enable change	• Increased positive parenting • Decreased coercive parenting • Improved parent-child relationships • Increased parental confidence	
Improved Parent Adjustment and Partner Relationships	• Help parents develop personal coping skills • Facilitate better communication between parenting partners	• Decreased parent stress, anxiety and depression • Decreased parental conflict • Improved marital satisfaction	
Improved Systems of Care	• Make program available in multiple formats • Deliver at a variety of locations that parents can access • Promote Peer Assisted Supervision and Support	• Improved communication amongst providers • Common language for parenting support • Less work in isolation • Increased access to parenting support • More efficiency in service delivery	
Healthier Communities	• Engage a wide variety of community partners	• Decreased child maltreatment • Decreased out-of-home placements • Decreased hospitalizations/ER visits • Strengthened parenting across community • Improvement in child behavior across community	

regarding which specific skills to include was based on a mix of clinical experience, research relating to teaching new skills and behaviors to children, and my own experience as a parent. I wanted to include all relevant skills that may be useful to parents in tackling a diverse range of problems. The logic model for the program appears in Table 7.2.

Challenges, Enablers, and Setbacks

Challenges

The main challenge was to develop the system over the next two decades (1993 to present) and to build an evidence base to support each component of the model. The research and development process underpinning Triple P required a sustained, long-term commitment to evolving the program. A small team of dedicated clinical researchers, who were former students of mine at UQ, undertook the task of developing the parenting resources for each program in the system. These resources included facilitators' manuals (including session guides and power point slides), parent workbooks, parenting tipsheets, and video material that demonstrated principles and techniques.

Other challenges addressed included:

Creating sufficient time to work on program development and dissemination. Many clinical academics with heavy teaching and supervision loads and limited grant funding find it challenging to allocate sufficient time to develop and test interventions. Securing competitive National Health and Medical Research Council and the Australian Research Council grant funding was essential to recruit staff to share the workload involved.

Identifying colleagues with a shared vision. I have worked with many very capable collaborators who shared the vision of creating a better world through positive parenting of children. This was a challenge initially when working in a psychiatry environment where most colleagues had different interests and used different theoretical models and approaches to treatment (psychodynamic, biomedical).

Securing institutional support. When we became serious about the dissemination of Triple P, we needed to secure institutional support. This included reaching agreement with the school, faculty, and senior executive regarding the management of the intellectual property vested in the program and a commercialization model that was acceptable to both program authors and the university. After reaching an agreement, the PFSC benefited from the support of successive heads of School of Psychology, Executive Deans of the Faculty, and senior university executives. This support included allocation of suitable research space, and three waves of strategic university funding to support the international growth of the program.

Changing the language of parent intervention. Over time, I became more critical of the language used in the field of parent training. Not all parents with problems with their children need "training," "therapy," or "treatment," particularly when programs are prevention focused and are delivered outside health care settings (e.g., schools, early childhood education settings, work places). I prefer the term "evidence-based parenting support" to reflect the wider range of effective prevention interventions. We sought to develop a "non-blaming" perspective in discussing parenting to reduce stigma and increase the social acceptability and desirability of participation in parenting programs. A non-blaming perspective assumes that all parents benefit from parenting support from time to time. To participate in a parenting program does not necessarily mean parents have skills deficits and need to be "trained" to alter dysfunctional behavior. Many parents have the skills but need to learn how to combine them with other skills to make a parenting plan work.

Setbacks

Setbacks included the turnover of key personnel, retaining suitable clinical research space, lack of infrastructure support, and financial pressures. A commitment to the overarching mission of promoting the well-being of children through good parenting, supported persistence in the face of setbacks, ensuring that setbacks were temporary and, where possible, were turned in to opportunities and learning. For example, concerns raised by social work colleagues about the value of Triple P with child protection clients in training programs led to the development of additional modules focused on parental attributions and anger management that were used with child protection cases.

Dealing with Critics

Critics of parenting programs based on social learning approaches have included those who identify themselves under the broad label of attachment theory, and increasingly trauma-informed therapy. Social learning theory based programs such as Triple P use contingent attention and rewards, and mild disciplinary consequences. At various times there have been influential articles in popular media claiming that the use of Time Out damages children's brains (Coyne, 2013; Siegal & Bryson, 2014). The absence of credible evidence to support such contentions has not diminished criticism of parenting interventions (Dadds & Tully, 2019). Our approach has been to emphasize the skills in Triple P that promote loving, secure, stable relationships between parents and children, and highlight evidence supporting the efficacy of programs that include specific disciplinary consequences such as Time Out and the almost complete absence of negative side effects when these procedures are employed correctly by parents (Morawska & Sanders 2011). Such views, when held by influential agency directors, can lead to an agency decision not to adopt Triple P. In each case we sought to counter such views by correcting misinformation (e.g., Triple P is only for well-educated, middle-class parents; Triple P does not address attachment). We developed a list of possible criticisms and included specific information in our "train the trainer" courses so that issues could be addressed directly in the training of professionals.

Major Influences

The formation of a purveyor organization (Triple P International Pty Ltd) dedicated to the dissemination of Triple P was a major milestone. It occurred at a time when there was no clear roadmap to follow about creating "one stop shop" implementation support for agencies using Triple P. As there were no directly relevant exemplars at the time for us to follow in developing a purveyor organization there was a lot of "trial and error" learning in the early years (1996 to 2001). TPI was formally licensed by UQ (the owners of the intellectual property vested in Triple P) in 2001. Over the past 20 years, TPI has become a medium sized business, and a significant employer of psychologists as contract trainers or implementation consultants.

Developing Program Content

Strategies for Developing Program Content

Program content for different variants of Triple P evolved by examining the existing theoretical and evidence base relating to specific child or parent problems, conducting epidemiological surveys of parents and practitioners to identify key needs and concerns, and identifying currently available "best practice" guidelines and evidence relating to what works. We identified examples of parenting situations that most parents with similar problems would relate to (e.g., problems with children following directions, sibling conflict, mealtime problems), and depicted these with realistic video footage of parents interacting with children and implementing parenting solutions with their children in those situations (e.g. descriptive praise, planned activities routines). Focus groups of parents and practitioners were conducted to check that problems selected, situations depicted, and solutions used were culturally appropriate and relevant to parents.

Development of Procedures for Training Trainers

The successful implementation of Triple P depends on having a trained and accredited workforce of professional trainers who can train other professionals to deliver Triple P to parents in different countries. As the Master trainer, I train a small number of carefully selected practitioners, mostly experienced Masters or PhD level psychologists, who have the potential to become accredited trainers for Triple P International with a colleague (Alan Ralph) in an initial six-day intensive training course. The training involves practitioners becoming familiar with all course materials (including video, presentations, participant notes, practitioner kits, and parent resources) used in different levels of the intervention and specific training exercises used to prepare practitioners to deliver the program.

Procedures for Training Professionals and for Maintaining Practitioner Fidelity

Triple P trainers are responsible for training practitioners typically in groups of 20 in different variants of the program. The curriculum for this training is the responsibility of the PFSC.

Procedures for Sustained Implementation

A major challenge for all evidence-based programs is to ensure practitioners are well trained, accredited, and properly supported by their employers as they implement the program over time. Table 7.3 links the theoretical basis of procedures with specific techniques used in Triple P and Table 7.4 provides a list of core professional competencies practitioners are introduced to in Triple P professional training courses.

An implementation framework based on the same self-regulation principles that underpin the Triple P approach to working with parents was developed

Table 7.3 Linkage between Theory and Intervention Procedures

Theoretical Perspectives	Influential Individuals	Procedures used Associated with Theory	Specific Procedures/Techniques Procedures
Applied Behavior Analysis	Todd Risley Ted Glynn	Direct observation Contingency analysis (SORK) Functional analysis Procedures to increase pro-social behavior Procedures to decrease problem behavior Programming for generalization	SORK analysis Teaching parent self-management skills Planned Activities Training in high risk settings *Developing positive relationship* • Brief quality time • Talking to children • Showing affection *Encouraging desirable behavior* • Descriptive praise • Giving positive attention • Providing engaging activities *Teaching new skills and behaviors* • Setting a good example • Using incidental teaching • Using ASK, SAY, DO • Using behavior charts *Managing misbehavior* • Establishing ground rules • Using directed discussion for rule breaking • Planned ignoring for minor problem behavior • Giving clear, calm instructions • Backing up instructions with logical consequences • Using quiet time for misbehavior • Using time out for serious misbehavior
Social Performance Theory	Gerald Patterson	Observation of parent-child interaction in the home	Identifying social learning influences (escalation traps, accidental rewards) maintain problem behavior Systematic assessment of outcomes Coaching and feedback
Cognitive social learning theory Coercion theory	Albert Bandura	Targeting cognitive mechanisms	Teaching parents self-regulation skills (self-determination of goals, self-monitoring, self-evaluation) Identifying attributions and cognitive biases Clarifying parental expectations of children and self

(Continued)

Table 7.3 (Continued) Linkage between Theory and Intervention Procedures

Theoretical Perspectives	Influential Individuals	Procedures used Associated with Theory	Specific Procedures/Techniques Procedures
Developmental theory	Betty Hart/ Todd Risley Burton White	Targeting language initiations of children	Using brief quality time for the incidental teaching of language Talking/listening to children Planning engaging activities to prevent problems
Public health/ Health promotion	Stanford Heart Disease Prevention Program	Targeting reducing/ increasing prevalence rates Parenting as a public health issue Prevention	Population level change in parenting as a target Use of multilevel interventions including media and low intensity intervention Parenting support for all parents (principle of "Proportionate universalism")

by Triple P International (McWilliam et al., 2016). The framework incorporates two key underlying principles of the Triple P system: minimal sufficiency and self-regulation. A multiphase process is used including initial engagement, commitment and contracting, implementation planning, training and accreditation, and finally implementation and maintenance. We also developed a PASS model of clinical supervision (peer assisted supervision and support) to promote fidelity and program use (Sanders & Murphy-Brennan, 2006). This approach to sustaining the professional quality of the workforce requires minimal resources on our part, and appears to encourage greater sustained engagement and dissemination: Providers who attend peer support sessions use Triple P more often with parents (Owens, Haskett & Norwalk, 2019).

Refining, Expanding, Disseminating

Refining Program Content and Modifying the Program

Triple P has continued to evolve and to respond to feedback from end-users, consumers, and new evidence relating to the effects of parenting and family relationships on developmental outcomes. Systematic inclusion of data collection procedures that solicit feedback from consumers has helped provide an evidence base to make decisions about what needs to change or requires refinement or adaptation of content and process of delivery. Feedback can relate to

Table 7.4 Core Professional Competencies Developed in Triple P Training Courses

Competency	Purpose	Benefits/Outcome
Setting up a conducive environment for parenting groups or individual consultations	To create a physical and emotional environment conducing to learning	Parents can focus on the content of sessions
Negotiating a clear session agenda	To provide structure of what is to be covered in a session	Parents understand what is required of them in each session and what will be covered
Using direct observations to conduct an excesses, deficits, assets analysis of a child or parents behavior	To identify potential goals for change	Targets and goals are appropriate and address factors contributing to the maintenance of problems
Selecting reliable and valid baseline assessment procedures	To ensure all relevant outcomes can be assessed before during and after intervention	Measures are sensitive to change due to the effects of intervention
Discussing causes of a child's behavior problem with an individual or group of parents	To assist parents recognizing the important role of parenting in causing or maintain problem behavior	Parents have a clear rationale for all parenting strategies introduced in Triple P
Demonstrating use of specific positive parenting skills	To ensure all practitioners know how to implement all procedures used in Triple P themselves	Practitioners can model all skills and can select examples that illustrate how skills are employed
Shaping parents use of parenting skills through constructive feedback	To ensure practitioners have the skills to assist parent change their parenting behavior	Practitioners can be supportive and can prompt and reinforce parents appropriately
Designing effective parenting strategies for high risk situations, such as when the parent is busy (e.g., on the phone) or under scrutiny from others (at the shops)	To ensure practitioners are able to apply parenting techniques in different situations	Procedures/techniques are use in a manner consistent with principles of effective usage
Helping parents set specific, actionable, age-appropriate change goals for their children	To ensure practitioners understand the importance of promoting self-regulation in parents	Parents take the lead in setting their own parenting goals
Dealing with resistance from parents within a group	To ensure common sources of resistance in groups is managed effectively	Legitimate concerns and queries from parents are addressed competently and confidently

(Continued)

Table 7.4 (Continued) Core Professional Competencies Developed in Triple P Training Courses

Competency	Purpose	Benefits/Outcome
Handling parents' questions about discipline	To ensure practitioners are aware of and can answer common questions about all procedures employed in Triple P	Parents misunderstanding are addressed in advance
Drawing from theory and empirical evidence in providing rationales	To ensure that parents know enough about underlying theory of positive parenting principles so they can apply this knowledge to new situations	Practitioners can use research to assist with answering parents questions
Using audiovisual equipment	To ensure that all equipment works and that practitioners can troubleshoot common equipment issues	AV equipment works, first time when it is needed with minimum of lost time because of problems
Giving parents homework assignments (e.g., reading tasks) to encourage self-directed learning	To make sure that between session practice tasks for parents are appropriate and like to be successful	Parents take the initiative in ensuring learning from sessions are implemented between sessions
Managing group process issues (disengagement, over talking)	To alert practitioners to common process issues that can contribute to groups running overtime	Practitioners confidently manage within session disruptions to learning
Helping parents set themselves realistic, specific goals for practice/behavior change	To ensure that practitioners facilitate parents taking control of their own goal setting	Parents when given the opportunity are active to generating solutions
Facilitating self-sufficiency by prompting parents to self-monitor and self-evaluate their performance through telephone consultations	To ensure parents do not become overly reliant of practitioners for solution to their parenting concerns	Parents are active learners, support each other
Referring families to appropriate agencies for further help if needed	To ensure practitioners know what to do if parents require more intensive or additional services	When appropriate parents are referred for additional support (financial concerns, serious mental health problems)

written materials (e.g., literacy level of tip sheets and workbooks), the quality of video examples, or the gender or ethnic mix of parents and children used in examples.

Promotion of Fidelity

Fidelity refers to the extent to which a program follows the protocol as outlined in the practitioner manual relevant to each intervention. It is useful to distinguish between content and process fidelity. To deliver a Triple P program with fidelity requires the practitioner to flexibly tailor their delivery to the needs of participating families or otherwise to risk drop out. The main concern is not with low risk variations, such as using different examples to those used in parent workbooks or videos, but with high risk variations, such as omitting a parenting strategy altogether (e.g., descriptive praise, time out) based on a practitioner's assumption that the approach is not suitable to a case. Another concern is adding a program component that is not part of Triple P (e.g., prayer, showing another video from a different program) and then representing it to parents as part of Triple P. In training, we encourage practitioners to use low risk variations as necessary and simultaneously discourage them from using high risk content or process variations. The rationale for avoiding high risk variations is that the program is being fundamentally changed, it decouples it from its evidence base, and is offering parents something different from what they understood they were agreeing to in making a commitment to participate in Triple P.

Sustainability Challenges

Sustaining the use of Triple P is more likely if agencies routinely collect outcome data about the family's experience of the program. When routine evidence is collected showing that the program works to produce meaningful results there is a strong incentive for practitioners and managers to continue to use a program. If outcomes achieved are poor or parents simply cannot be engaged, the program it is unlikely to survive. All agencies using Triple P are encouraged to evaluate outcomes. Clear rationales are provided to agency leads and all participating staff. Specific measures and tools are recommended for every level of the program.

Innovation and New Program Variants

Since the initial development of the program, numerous innovations have taken place. These innovations have resulted in the development of different delivery modalities (e.g., group, online, over the phone, use of mass media), program variants for specific populations (e.g., parents of gifted and talented children, children with feeding problems, anxiety problems), and cultural adaptations for Indigenous parents. Program variants were developed for specific child- or family-challenges. For example, Stepping Stones Triple P was developed for parents of children with developmental disabilities.

The Crucial Role of a Purveyor Organization for Dissemination

One important aspect of scaling a program is for the program developer to have secured the intellectual property that comprises the intervention. In the case of Triple P, all contributing authors assigned their intellectual property rights to the University of Queensland so that the program can be licensed via the University's major technology transfer company to a third party purveyor organisation, Triple P International Pty Ltd. This assignment facilitated the program being disseminated worldwide, which would not have been possible without first securing the intellectual property rights of the program. We needed a "one stop shop" to manage all aspects of disseminating and scaling the program. This involved coordinating the publishing of written materials, production of video and web based programs, the marketing of Triple P, and providing professional training and implementation support to agencies using Triple P. To create an economically sustainable model for dissemination, Triple P International was established as a start-up company and granted a perpetual license by the University of Queensland to disseminate Triple P worldwide. At the time in 1997, we were unable to find any traditional academic publishers prepared to take on all of the functions outlined above so that the purveyor organization could run an efficient dissemination operation on a global scale. The guiding operational principle we evolved for Triple P was that all programs in the Triple P system needed to have an evidence base that justified their inclusion. The intellectual property invested in the program remained under the PFSC's control until sufficient evidence was available showing that the program variant worked. At that point, programs were offered through the license agreement to TPI to disseminate and they had the right of first refusal to decide if they wished to publish the program. Most programs that have an evidence base have been disseminated by TPI, though all programs selected must be considered commercially viable.

Managing Conflicts of Interest (COI)

When program developers are involved in the evaluation of programs, an unavoidable conflict of interest occurs that needs to be managed. Problems with lack of transparency arise where developers do not routinely disclose their COI to journal editors, and must be internally managed by universities as part of research integrity policies. Strategies such as preregistering trials, provision of original data, increased use of open source journals, use of independent clinical trial statisticians to conduct analyses, and the removal of the developer from the data interpretation reduce the risk of bias. These steps have gone some way in reducing the risk of bias intervention research; however, it does not eliminate the problem completely. We have developed specific guidelines for developers regarding the management of COI (Sanders, Kirby, Toumborou, Carey & Havighurt, 2019).

Going to Scale

With the internet and the development of a global market, working internationally has become more common. However, there are still major challenges relating to the costs of quality language translations of parent and training materials, importation of foreign goods and services, application of relevant taxation law, slow speed of the internet in some parts of the world making video conferencing unreliable, and the logistics of working in different time zones. While these problems are not insurmountable they should not be underestimated either.

Barriers (Policies, Funding of Research, and Services)

The main obstacle to the dissemination of Triple P is a lack of policy commitment to implement evidence-based parenting support programs. The responsibilities for parenting interventions are generally uncoordinated, being dispersed across many departments, disciplines, and services. Parenting support often seems to be "everyone's business but no one's responsibility". Such a situation can lead to lack of accountability, poor coordination of services, underfunding, overlapping responsibilities, major gaps in service provision, and uncoordinated and inefficient delivery of services.

Lessons Learned

Building Meaningful Collaborations and Long-term Relationships

To ensure evidence-based programs have a life beyond an initial demonstration trial, developers need to give careful attention to the environment of potential adoption of the intervention. Programs are more likely to be implemented if they have a good "ecological fit" to the delivery context, system, and population that they are designed for. Several steps can be put in place to increase the contextual relevance of a program before initial trialing, including: (1) The establishment of a professional and scientific advisory body to provide feedback about the planned intervention; (2) establishing an end-user reference group. End-user groups that include professionals working with a defined parent population bring a unique perspective to the research and development process. This includes their views on participant burden, clarity, clinical utility, and cultural relevance of examples used to illustrate principles and teaching points, perceived effectiveness, and implementation challenges of strategies advocated, and barriers and facilitators for engaging and maintaining involvement of parents; (3) parent focus groups can feed back and generate ideas on cultural acceptability and relevance of an intervention (including methods of recruiting and engaging parents); and (4) a plan for ensuring that program delivery will be funded. Having a training budget to train staff without having a corresponding allocation of resources to enable a program to be implemented by practitioners makes it much more difficult to sustain implementation over time. Local arrangements will vary depending on country, state or province, and jurisdiction.

Responding to Cultural Diversity

Our group has developed a Collaborative Partnership and Adaption Model (C-PAM) for ensuring parenting interventions had a good cultural fit for Indigenous parents in Australia (Turner, Sanders, McKeown, and Shepherd, 2018). This model involved the use of focus groups of parents, practitioners, and elders to review an existing evidence-based practice to identify what program components needed to be retained or adapted to ensure the program was suitable for Indigenous parents. An RCT tested the efficacy and cultural acceptability of the discussion group Triple P intervention (level 3) with Maori parents of preschool aged children. The trial demonstrated that the culturally-adapted intervention was both effective in reducing children's disruptive behavior, and was also considered highly culturally appropriate by participants (Keown, Sanders, Shepherd, & Franke, 2018). A similar approach can be used with other diverse groups to link culturally-based values to Triple P principles and techniques.

Developing and Revising High Quality Program Resources

To ensure that programs remain relevant to the needs of parents, financial resources and time need to be set aside to "refresh" program materials periodically. Video footage can date quickly. Also the means of showing it changes as new techniques of presenting information evolve, and technology changes. We keep all video material under constant review. Some examples seem timeless and continue to have relevance for successive generations of parents, while other footage dates. However, modern parents raised themselves in an age of technology also have much higher expectations relating to the production value of program materials used. For example, their children may be involved in some amazing school projects that include sophisticated multimedia presentations that can make some experienced program developers look like amateurs.

Importance of Market Considerations and Policy Context

The extent to which a program is viewed as having "market" potential for dissemination is determined by multiple factors. Market potential is an estimate of the maximum sales of a product or service during a certain period. It is an estimate as it assumes that you can capture the entire market for a product. Factors we considered include how prevalent a problem is, how much of a concern, and how costly it is to government, whether there is an available workforce to deliver the program, the time and costs of program delivery, the costs to government of not intervening, the extent to which there is consumer demand for the program, and whether the implementation of a solution is a government policy priority. Each of these considerations needs to be factored into decisions to develop, test, and disseminate a new intervention. Changes of government, stated priorities, and the health of the economy can improve or worsen the funding support available to implement an intervention. Market research to gauge the likely "pull demand" from parents as consumers is desirable.

Importance of Policy Advocacy and Understanding the Drivers of Change

Many program developers/clinical researchers struggle to get their innovations noticed by funding decision-makers. Clinical researchers need to develop more sophisticated methods of advocating for the adoption of evidence-based practices: Greater attention to the time lines associated with government policy commitments and announcements, the appropriate conveying of important policy relevant research findings to policy makers, and the use of others to advocate for programs (e.g., professional associations, public affairs lobbyists, champions, consumers). Program developers can find it difficult to advocate for their own programs and are often concerned about being viewed as self-serving and as having unavoidable conflicts of interest. We have found it is generally better to advocate for all evidence-based programs addressing a particular problem than exclusively to focus on one's own program in isolation.

Being Nimble and Responding to Opportunities

Innovation is often opportunistic in the sense that a particular set of events occurs that requires government action and a funding response (e.g., Commissions of Inquiry into the Abuse of Children in Care). These funding opportunities can provide a context for the adoption of evidence-based programs.

The Challenges of Working with Organizations that Manage "Evidence-based" Lists

Evidence-based lists are maintained by several organizations to provide advice and guidance to governments, agencies, and commissioners of service about what interventions work. Such lists vary in quality and rigor of the review process for programs (e.g., Blueprints for Prevention, Early Intervention Foundation). Unfortunately, there is not a high degree of agreement amongst the various lists in different countries reviewing the same evidence.

Expecting the Unexpected

Even the very best practices can be disrupted by unforeseen and largely uncontrollable events. These include unexpected defunding of or reductions in funding available to agencies delivering evidence-based parenting programs stemming from changes in government priorities. A change of government or Minister can result in different priorities that differentiate new political leadership from the previous administration (e.g., having greater focus on preventing youth suicide versus early intervention and prevention). The loss of key influential champions of parenting programs (e.g., due to promotion, retirement, ill health) can mean loss of political support for a program. Highly restrictive work practices can prevent staff delivering parenting programs in evenings or weekends. The global economy and disadvantageous currency fluctuations when training in other countries can create unexpected financial pressures. Some agencies experience "innovation fatigue" where staff believe they are expected to change safe, familiar, but often non-evidence based work practices; staff can become cynical and undermine the change process. These events are not peculiar to parenting programs. However, they require strong leadership, passionate commitment to the cause, and sufficient emotional resilience to avoid reaching the conclusion that this is "all too hard."

Future Directions

Evidence based programs such as Triple P must continue to evolve to remain relevant to the contemporary needs of parents and communities.

Moving Beyond the Prevention of Mental Health Problems and Child Maltreatment

Much of the parenting literature has focused on the reduction of disruptiveness, aggression, and, to a lesser extent, anxiety. To date, relatively little attention has been devoted to the development of pro-sociality in children. Such an approach would entail identifying specific positive attributes that parenting could promote in children.

Tackling "Wicked" Problems of Global Significance

We recently argued that parenting programs have a potentially very important role to play in tackling major environmental problems. Simmons and

Sanders (2018) presented an example of such an approach by showing that villagers in an Indonesian coastal village in Salliyer could be trained to adopt more ecologically friendly practices in disposal of plastic waste rather than deposit waste into rivers and waterways, which, in turn, damaged coastal reefs and fish stock. The intervention *My Future, My Oceans* (Simmons & Sanders, 2018) used two brief group intervention sessions based on the self-regulation model of Triple P to target increasing awareness of environment destruction, and when compared to a control village post training there was a significant increase in appropriate disposal and recycling of plastic waste.

Targeting the United Nations Sustainable Development Goals

The above illustration shows the potential of parenting interventions in targeting the family unit and thereby increasing personal and family agency to address other sustainable development goals including but not restricted to ending poverty, promoting healthy lifestyles, achieving gender equity, and reducing climate change (Sanders, Divan, Singhal, Turner, Velleman, Michelson & Patel, under review).

Addressing Parental Trauma and Historical Adverse Childhood Experiences (ACEs)

Although many parents with histories of adversity in their own childhood have participated in Triple P interventions, some parents have an accumulation of risk factors that goes beyond child abuse and neglect and may include other risk exposures such as growing up in a household with a parent who has a history of mental illness or substance use, incarceration, family violence, or marital breakdown. A self-regulation approach when first applied to parenting concerns can also be applied to other adult concerns including coping with stress, relationship conflict, attributional biases and depression, and inadequate self-care. We are currently testing a 10-session Family Life Skills Triple P intervention that blends targeting parenting and other life skills with parents who have a history of high levels of ACEs.

Using Artificial Intelligence (AI) to Enhance the Quality of Professional Training in Evidence-based Parenting Interventions

A major barrier to the widespread implementation of evidence-based parenting interventions is the costs of professional training, particularly outside metropolitan areas. Artificial Intelligence (AI) or learning machines offers the prospect of providing learning experiences and opportunities to train practitioners at lower costs and higher efficiency than existing training, which requires the practitioner to take two to five days away from their workplace, depending on the course. A specific challenge for designers of future AI training courses is to develop functional equivalent learning experiences to the coaching procedures currently employed. These typically involve practitioners observing and role playing skills, receiving feedback from peers or instructor, and repeating until they master it. There is no functional equivalent to well-timed feedback that specifically addresses the timing, sequencing, and effective tone of a practitioner's interaction with a client, although self-evaluation can also be useful.

Conclusion

After four decades of research and development, the Triple P system continues to evolve. It has been supported by a thriving research culture and explicit knowledge exchange process that bring together researchers, disseminators, practitioners, policy makers, and consumers. We will have reached an important milestone when accessible, high quality, and culturally informed parenting programs are embedded into the social fabric of communities. With significant investment in population-based parenting support programs, many children and adolescents will achieve their true potential, and society as a whole will benefit from it.

References

Ballard, K. D., & Glynn, T. (1975). Behavioral self-management in story writing with elementary school children 1. *Journal of Applied Behavior Analysis*, 8(4), 387–398. doi: 10.1901/jaba.1975.8-387

Bandura, A., & Walters, R. H. (1977). *Social learning theory*, 1. Englewood Cliffs, NJ: Prentice-Hall.

Coyne, J. (2013). Parenting from the outside-in: Reflections on parent training during a potential paradigm shift. *Australian Psychologist*, 48(5), 379–387. doi: 10.1111/ap.12010

Dadds, M. R., & Tully, L. A. (2019). What is it to discipline a child: What should it be? A reanalysis of time-out from the perspective of child mental health, attachment, and trauma. *American Psychologist*. Retrieved from https://psycnet.apa.org/doi/10.1037/amp0000449

Day, J. J., & Sanders, M. R. (2018). Do parents benefit from help when completing a self-guided parenting program online? A randomized controlled trial comparing Triple P Online with and without telephone support. *Behavior Therapy*, 49(6), 1020–1038. https://doi.org/10.1 016/j.beth.2018.03.002

Keown, L. J., Sanders, M. R., Franke, N. & Shepherd, M. (2018). Te Whānau Pou Toru: A randomized controlled trial (RCT) of a culturally adapted low-intensity variant of the Triple P-Positive Parenting Program for indigenous Māori families in New Zealand. *Prevention Science*, 19(7), 954–965. https://doi.org/10.1007/s11121-018-0886-5

McWilliam, J., Brown, J., Sanders, M. R., & Jones, L. (2016). The Triple P implementation framework: The role of purveyors in the implementation and sustainability of evidence-based programs. *Prevention Science*, 17(5), 636–645.

Morawska, A., & Sanders, M. R. (2006). Self-administered behavioral family intervention for parents of toddlers: Part 1. Efficacy. *Journal of Consulting and Clinical Psychology, 74*(1), 10–19. doi.org/10.1037/0022-006X.74.1.10

Morawska, A., & Sanders, M. R. (2011). Parental use of time out revisited: A useful or harmful parenting strategy? *Journal of Child and Family Studies, 20*(1), 1–8. doi: 10.1007/s10826-010-9371-x

Owens, C. R., Haskett, M. E., & Norwalk, K. (2019). Peer assisted supervision and support and providers' use of Triple P- Positive Parenting Program. *Journal of Child and Family Studies, 28*, 1664–1672. doi: 10.1007/s10826-019-01385-w

Patterson, G. R., Reid, J. B., Jones, R. R., & Conger, R. E. (1975). *A social learning approach to family intervention: Families with aggressive children* (vol. 1). Castalia Publishing Company.

Sanders, M. R., Baker, S., & Turner, K. M. (2012). A randomized controlled trial evaluating the efficacy of Triple P Online with parents of children with early-onset conduct problems. *Behaviour Research and Therapy, 50*(11), 675–684. doi: 10.1016/j.brat.2012.07.004

Sanders, M. R., Divan, G., Singhal, M., Turner, K. M. T., Velleman, R., Michelson, D., & Patel, V. (under review). Scaling up parenting interventions is critical for attaining the sustainable development goals.

Sanders, M. R., & Glynn, T. (1981). Training parents in behavioral self-management: An analysis of generalization and maintenance. *Journal of Applied Behavior Analysis, 14*(3), 223–237. doi: 10.1901/jaba.1981.14-22.

Sanders, M. R., Kirby, J. N., Toumbourou, J. W., Carey, T. A., & Havighurst, S. S. (2019). Innovation, research integrity, and change: A conflict of interest management framework for program developers. *Australian Psychologist, 55*(2), 91–101. doi: 10.1111/ap.12404

Sanders, M. R., & Mazzucchelli, T. G. (2018). *The power of positive parenting: Transforming the lives of children, parents and communities using the Triple P system.* New York: Oxford University Press.

Sanders, M. R., & Murphy-Brennan, M. (2006). *Peer assisted supervision and support: A practice guide.* Brisbane, QLD: Triple P international.

Siegel, D. J., & Bryson, T. P. (2014, September 23). 'Time-outs' are hurting your child. *TIME.*

Simmons, K., & Sanders, M. R. (2018). *My future, my oceans.* Brisbane, QLD: Parenting and Family Support Centre, The University of Queensland.

Turner, K. M., Sanders, M. R., Keown, L. J., & Shepherd, M. (2018). A collaborative partnership adaptation model. In M. R. Sanders & T. G. Mazzuchelli (Eds.), *The power of positive parenting: Transforming the lives of children, parents, and communities using the Triple P system* (pp. 310–320). New York: Oxford University Press.

Part III

Family

Chapter 8

The Development of the Strengthening Families Program for 10 to 14 Year Olds

Eugenia Hartsook and Virginia Molgaard

Starting Point

On a spring morning many years ago, Virginia Molgaard received a phone call that changed her life. Her husband was teaching in a small college on the shores of Lake Michigan and she had taken a few years off from teaching music in public school to raise their two young daughters. Her older brother and his wife had been killed by a young drunk driver. In the grief and chaos of the following days, they thought about who would raise their four children, ages 3 to 13. After consulting with a psychologist who knew the family, friends who were social workers, and with much prayer, they decided to take in the children. They made some minor housing adjustments and very soon were a family of eight, instead of four. Two of the orphaned children, the three-year-old boy and the eight-year-old girl had special needs. Soon they were working with social workers and psychiatrists to find ways to meet their needs. After some unsuccessful attempts at family therapy, Virginia decided to return to graduate school in psychology and family studies to learn more about families in crisis and to learn how best to help all six children deal with the upheaval.

At the end of Virginia's Masters and Ph.D. degrees she was invited to join the faculty at Iowa State University and was offered a position at the new family research institute. It was a fitting position because a group of researchers there had been studying the effects of the rural economic crisis on families. There she worked with Dr. Richard Spoth and colleagues to write a grant to the National Institute of Mental Health to develop and test a substance use prevention curriculum for young adolescents and their families in economically stressed areas. The plan was to create a program with separate components for parents and children, as well as time in each session for the family as a whole.

Strategy and Theory of Change

When someone takes the time and energy to write a program to help meet the needs of some group, he or she wants it to be successful. That means that people will come to the program and be persuaded and taught to change attitudes and/or behavior to meet a need or improve their lives in some way. It is not enough for a youth or family to simply attend the first session; rather one must pay attention, perhaps learn some new ways of thinking or acting, and return for the next session. The participants must believe it is worth their time and effort. This section describes some of the principles that helped guide the program into something worthwhile.

One of the most important principles is that all people and families have strengths. Program participants should be encouraged to build on their strengths. Presenting a strength-based approach begins at recruitment. Make sure those you wish to recruit do not see this as a program for "youth at risk" or "troubled" families. Instead use words like, "Come to this program to help your child have a successful time in the teen years" and "Have fun and learn together with your child". In working with adults, for example, participants' different views and situations should be respected while, at the same time, participants should be encouraged to try a variety of effective parenting tools.

Using an approach based on strengths helps in several ways. If either a young person or adult feels put down when they share something or answer a question, they are much less willing to participate or even continue to attend. If people have had a positive experience, including respect for and from other participants, it can be a powerful factor in the ability to recruit in the future because they are trusted voices of the community. An example of using the strength approach in the Strengthening Families Program: 10–14 can be found in one of the very few worksheets in the parent session. Parents rate the degree to which they use a number of positive parenting tools (seldom, sometimes, or often) and mark things they might like to improve. No one except the parent sees his or her responses.

A related idea is that all participants should have a pleasant and fun experience. It takes a great deal of dedication, for example, for parents and children to come week after week for seven, two-hour sessions. One mother shared at the end of a program evening, "I was so tired after work I wanted to skip tonight but my son said we had to go because it was so much fun." Over the years, numerous positive comments have been shared by facilitators, parents, and young people about what a good time families have in SFP 10–14. Part of the fun we have observed in parent sessions was adults enjoying sharing their own frustrations and problems with other caregivers who had similar experiences. We have also observed parents and children laughing together and becoming closer as a family. It cannot be emphasized enough how important it is for participants in a program to have a fun experience (Achor, 2011). Positive and happy feelings make it more likely that people will pay attention, be committed to positive change, and apply the learning in their everyday life.

Using an active learner style of teaching was also important in the development of this program. Think of the many conferences with presentations by researchers and practitioners that you have attended. Some presentations were probably hard to follow and boring. A few hours after the presentation it might have been difficult to remember the content, let alone apply it. However, other presentations were likely engaging, creating the feeling that the new information would be useful on a practical basis. This type of learning often involves interaction, for example the presenter asking for participants' thoughts and ideas. The presenter then continues to ask probing questions to delve more deeply into the issues, adding ideas and suggestions that no one has mentioned, or expanding on one of their ideas from time to time. With this approach participants feel included and empowered instead of overwhelmed with information that might or might not be helpful.

An important guideline used in creating this program was the belief that most people do not think in the abstract when it comes to issues about relationships, behavior, and values. Instead, they think about real life situations and experiences. Therefore, a program should include concrete examples from everyday life, showing positive ways of interacting, and not-so-good ways. Using terms that are familiar and giving everyday examples make it more likely that people will be motivated to change attitudes and behavior. When a program seems more academic and "bookish", most people are turned off and it is less likely that they will be engaged and listen to what is presented.

There are several guiding thoughts about some practical considerations when creating a curriculum. Programs used within agencies and communities are likely to include people of various abilities and reading levels. For that reason, all worksheets and handouts for adults were written at the eighth-grade reading level. Another consideration was the use of specific words to designate participants, for example, parent and child. Parenting is done by many people other than parents: grandparents, aunts and uncles, foster parents, even an older sibling. For that reason, we use the term, "caregiver". Especially in the youth sessions, using the term "parent" is likely to make a child who is not being raised by his or her parent feel different or left out. The word you use for the young people in the program is important also. As they become older, many youth dislike being referred to as "children" and so in the materials the term "youth", as well as "young people" is used. It is important to consider these wording issues as you interact with participants and create printed material.

A strong emphasis during Virginia's graduate work had been on Family Systems, the theory that explains how any issue that affects even one member of the family, has an effect on everyone (Kerr, 2000). In terms of substance use prevention, Family Systems Theory would say that all attitudes and behaviors in the family affect each family member's use of substances. Therefore, to help young people avoid problems with substances, parents, as well as the young people themselves, should be involved. When this program was written there were a number of prevention programs for children or for parents, but they had limited effectiveness. Very few curricula worked with both adults and children, and none were designed for children between the ages of 10 and 14.

That period of early adolescence is a particularly challenging period for both parents and children. Many parents fear the upcoming independence of their children and by this age some have already noticed changes in their children that are concerning, such as spending more time alone and sharing less with the parents. Children themselves also face challenges including rapidly changing bodies and emotions, new pressures from peers, and negotiating a new school with older youth. Aware of the challenges at this age, we viewed it as vital to commit to creating a program that reached both children and parents. Because of this, the Strengthening Families Program has family sessions, where they can practice the skills they learned in separate sessions.

Creating Content

In the past, people often developed programs with a common-sense approach, choosing topics and activities they thought were important or necessary for a particular population. Little attention was given to studying what researchers in the particular field had discovered about the issue. By the mid-90s, funders at the state and federal level reached the conclusion that they did not want to give grants to groups who were not making use of the latest research to develop their programs. They began to search for "best practices" curricula that had made use of findings from research and that could be shown to produce positive outcomes for individuals and families. This was the setting when Virginia began to author this program.

Virginia's first step in creating content was to find out what the risk and protective factors are for the issue being addressed. For example, we learned that there are several factors that predict early use of substances like alcohol and other drugs, including attitudes and behavior of young people themselves as well as their parents. Her next step was to determine which of the risk factors for the particular problem could be influenced by a program. After she identified several risk or protective factors for the problem the program would address, she broke down each risk factor into several more specific issues. For example, knowing that harsh parenting puts young people at risk of substance use, Virginia asked herself what components of harsh parenting she could address. Virginia decided to focus on teaching parents to have realistic rules based on their child's age and development; using a kind, non-critical tone of voice; and administering appropriate consequences that reflect the severity of the misbehavior rather than the parent's level of anger (e.g., taking away screen time for half an hour, not a whole evening, for a minor misbehavior).

The last step in creating content was to develop specific ways of teaching the concepts that are interactive and use concrete examples from everyday life. Virginia used several teaching strategies, such as: (1) Brainstorming: Participants are asked to offer examples of rules that are and are not appropriate for a 12-year-old child. (2) Role play: Participants and facilitators role play examples of parents speaking in a harsh or critical voice, and then the group is asked to consider what a child in that situation might feel and what the results might be. (3) Break-out discussion: Participants gather in pairs or small groups to discuss consequences that are appropriate and ones that are too harsh, and then share their ideas with the whole group.

After the program was written and before it was tested, the materials were shared with schools where it would be conducted to solicit feedback from local stakeholders. A school principal asked the question, "How will you know whether the outcome will be due to the skills of the particular facilitators or due to the effectiveness of the program itself?" Then she suggested, "Why don't you make videotapes for the parent sessions with the program's content? Then you will know that each group receives the same information." Virginia had not considered using videotapes, but as soon as the suggestion was made, she knew that it would be an excellent way of building fidelity. When a program is being tested it is important that each group receives the "same" program and is not unduly affected by the skills of each particular facilitator. This is a definition of "fidelity". In addition, it would be easier for participants to remember and internalize the dynamics of "real life" families in video scenes than long verbal descriptions.

The material written for facilitators to present in the parent sessions was then turned into scripts for video narrators to deliver. Role plays were created for actors showing common family situations between parents and children, as well as typical conversations parents might have with each other about parenting concerns. They were based on experiences found to be common in research and in life. The wording reflected those that families' use when speaking to each other, more casual and more emotional. After the scripts and role plays were written, videographers were used to film both the narrations and the role plays. Using videotapes helped meet two goals: avoiding long lectures by facilitators and showing concrete examples of ineffective and effective interactions between family members. Each video for the parent sessions is about 15 minutes long, and includes role plays of typical family scenes as well as narrators who present information. The rest of the session is spent discussing the video, examples from personal experience, and translating the new understanding into everyday applications for their own families. A similar approach was taken for the two youth sessions that taught youth what to say to handle peer pressure situations and also in two family sessions demonstrating family meetings and parents helping their children remember how to handle peer pressure. Using videos for some of the sessions also made the program easier to teach. This early refinement of using videos contributed to several goals of the program—using concrete examples from real life, maintaining fidelity, and promoting participant enjoyment.

The original program was piloted in an economically disadvantaged rural community. These youth did not represent young people in more urban and diverse communities. Because of this, Virginia met with colleagues who had experience working with all kinds of youth in many settings. Together they developed creative games that taught the same material, but in a more engaging way. For example, in Youth Session Four, the original program had a discussion about common rules young people have and what negative things might happen when they break a rule (e.g., cheating on a test in school or going someplace they were not supposed to). This was developed into the Driving Game. In this game each youth gets to pretend they can already drive. There are stations set up around the room that create an itinerary for the "drivers" including a Driver's License Station, their home, their friend's home, a soccer game, a movie, and finally, the pizza place. As the game proceeds, players draw a card at each place that tells whether they followed the rule and drove safely. If they followed the rule they proceed to the next place. If they broke a rule or talked back to their parent, they lost a turn and had to stay where they were. They experience consequences in a simulated "real life" situation rather than just talking about the value of rules. The activity ends with each child describing the rules they had followed or broken and the consequences they experienced. They have fun and learn at the same time.

In family sessions, both adults and young people have a chance to practice the skills they are learning in their own separate sessions and build family connections. In most of the family sessions parents and children are working together in their own family unit, having specific discussions that are designed to encourage sharing and bring family members closer together. There are also large group games and activities.

In the following description, you can see an example of how the parent, youth, and family sessions are a unified whole. The first youth session focuses on encouraging youth to think about the kind of future they want. The activity includes a broader picture of the future than simply what kind of job they might want to have. Each child also thinks about domains of their future life: what they might like to do with friends and family, what hobbies they would like, and how they will stay strong and healthy. To make this more engaging and concrete for the youth, Virginia and her colleagues created the idea of Treasure Maps. Each child creates a Treasure Map by using magazine clippings as well as words and drawings to answer the above questions. The name "Treasure Map" was used to encourage children to think of their future as a treasure, something valuable.

At the end of the first parent session, there is an activity that illustrates for the parents that even though youth at this age may have dreams for the future that are probably not very realistic, it is important to support their goals. Research shows that young people do better during the teen years if they believe that they have a positive future. Caregivers are encouraged to be supportive as children talk about their dreams for the future, even if they are unrealistic.

Next, in the family session the children's "Treasure Maps" are displayed (without names) and parents try to guess which map was created by their own child. After each parent has found his or her child's map, they sit down together so that they can have a conversation about what the child hopes for in the future. Then parents practice helping their child think of things they could do right now to begin to move towards their goals. For example, if a son wants to be in professional sports, he needs to do things right now to be strong and healthy and keep his grades up so he can be on the school team. In the last part of the activity, the parents and children each have a set of simple questions to ask the each other. The child asks his or her parent(s) questions about what life was like for the parent(s) when they were young—what their goals were and what did they did for fun. In a closing circle (described below), everyone brings Treasure Maps and each child and caregiver shares with the group one of the goals on the map.

In addition to creating content for the family sessions, it was important to think about the logistics of how the sessions would flow. In this program the first hour is spent with caregivers and youth in separate rooms for their activities. After the separate sessions, the children join their parents who have been meeting in a space large enough for the whole group to be together for the family session. To alleviate chaos as the groups come together for the family session, each family session starts with a group game which the facilitators have explained while everyone is still in the separate groups. As the children come into the room, facilitators help children join their own caregivers and move into the game space.

One thing learned early on was the importance of a closing circle activity with all the families together. During the pilot it was discovered that the closing circle keeps families wanting to be involved until the end of the session instead of having some families want to leave early because it provides closure and allows participants to learn more about each other. During the closing circle there is a poster with a prepared statement for each person to share with the group. For example, after family session two each parent says, "One of my child's strengths is…" and each child says, "One of my parent's strengths is…". After everyone has shared, the children say together the creed that they learned in their own session, "We are strong young people with a great future. We are making good decisions, so we reach our goals." Then the parents say theirs, "We are strong and caring parents who show love and set limits. We are helping our children become responsible young adults." The session ends with the whole group repeating the family creed, "We are strong families who care about each other and have fun together." The creeds were developed based on the program's goals and as a way to provide positive affirmations. The closing circle serves three purposes. Firstly, it reinforces the learning from the family session. Secondly, it creates a strong sense of community within the group. Finally, it creates a friendly and organized ending to the evening.

Refining, Expanding, Dissemination

After the first part of the research was complete, Extension Family Life Specialist staff from seven areas in Iowa were trained. They conducted the program in both rural and urban sites over the next several years, with good results. As the research continued with the original families completing six-month, one year, and two-year follow up questionnaires, it was hoped that the program would soon be carried out beyond Iowa. By the time of the two-year follow-up, the research showed that the program was very successful in reducing youth substance use and aggression, increasing positive skills for parents, and building supportive family interactions. The program was listed on national websites such as the Center for Substance Use Prevention (CSAP), the Office of Juvenile Justice and Delinquency Prevention (OJJDP), and the US Department of Education, as a "best practices" curriculum, shown to be successful in randomized, controlled studies. Soon requests for training from local organizations around the country began to come.

As the requests came in from groups with diverse racial and ethnic families, it became apparent that the videotapes had to be re-done. The initial research project was done in all-white communities and the actors in the videos were white, while the narrators were African-American as well as white. Videos were now needed that represented diverse families. Through local grant funding, the videos were revised using African-American, Hispanic, and Asian actors.

The visual aspect of the manual was also revised. A new format with two columns on each page, which would be even easier for facilitators to use, was created. In the new format, the left-hand column of each page included instructions for facilitators such as: *(1) Process questions on the video screen and encourage discussion. (2) Pass out parent/caregiver worksheet and circulate to offer help. (3) Remind them that all of us do some things well and we could improve on things.* It also includes samples of flip chart lists for activities in which participants are sharing suggestions and ideas. In parent sessions, the right-hand column has the script for the video tape with both narrator parts and role play dialogues. This allows for the possible situation in which the video equipment is not working for a particular session. In the youth sessions, the right-hand column is used for diagrams, game layouts, and short suggestions for brainstorming and running the learning games.

The program was developed at Iowa State University and they handled the sale and distribution of the revised leader guides, videotapes, and supporting materials. There was no mechanism at the university for training facilitators outside of Iowa, so Virginia, along with her husband, who had been involved in the original teaching and research, used vacation days to conduct trainings outside of the state. After a few years, the requests were too numerous for them to handle, so they set up several training teams with people who had taught the program in the initial research project and were experienced facilitators. An important step was developing so that there would be fidelity in training as well as in actual community implementation of the program. Two trainers would work together during the training for the 21 sessions of the program (seven parent, seven youth, and seven family sessions). During the early stage of national training, a two-day training agenda was used. It was soon realized that in order for new facilitators to be prepared to lead groups and not be overwhelmed by the amount of content, the training time needed to expand to three days. In the training, participants experience each activity in each session from the point of view of the participant. For example, during the youth sessions, trainees are asked to assume the role of youth attending the program and they go through each activity as it would be done in a real group of youth. By the end of the training, the new facilitators will have experienced the program in much the same way that families will during an actual program implementation in the community. This allows the facilitators to better understand how to clarify directions and be prepared for possible participant questions.

The topic of family recruitment deserves special consideration. Recruitment is the hardest when the program is being offered for the first time in an agency or community. It is best to find and inform a group of six to eight people, who are known and respected in the community from the target audience to assist in recruitment. For example, if you wish to run a program in a school for parents of sixth graders, invite some parents whose children are in that grade to attend a short meeting to introduce the program and gather some enthusiasm. Describe the purpose of the program and show some examples of fun activities and projects within the program. Ask them for ideas on how to get the word out and see if each of them would be willing to invite some families. Let them know that the program will build on the strengths they already have and show parenting tools that might help them with their own children. After the program has been offered successfully even one time, have a meeting with adult participants who came to the program and found it helpful and fun. They will be your best help in recruiting people the next time you run the program, both by word of mouth and perhaps by inviting specific families. In both groups offer refreshments if possible.

Take photos of activities and family discussions to use in recruitment, if the families agree to have their photos used in recruitment activities and print material. Send a photo with a description of the recent program to your local print and web-based media outlets to spread the word. Use photos of scenes during the program in which youth or families are engaging in a fun game or activity. Create a simple flier to advertise the program using a few photos and some positive comments from actual participants, such as, "We learned how important is to spend time together as a family" and "I learned what to say if I'm getting peer pressured."

It is also important to be aware of the wrong kind of recruitment that can be stigmatizing. During one training, it was emphasized that it was a strength-based program for all kinds of families. A minister who was very excited about the program, attended the training. Later, when asked how the program was going he said, "I couldn't get anyone to come." When asked how he recruited, he said he tried everything; announcing from the pulpit, putting up fliers, writing about it in the newsletter. When asked how he described the program he said, "We have a great new program for families at risk."

Lessons Learned

An overarching lesson that we have learned in developing SFP, as well as in working with others in adapting the program in specific ways, is the importance of integrity in claims of originality and ownership. Although it is useful to draw ideas for program development from discussions with colleagues and existing program curricula, it is also critical to maintain integrity of authorship. It is always important for authors to ask themselves if their activities are truly original: Programs can be based on the same theories, but how those ideas are made concrete must be unique.

We have also learned lessons in training facilitators around managing their concerns. For example, facilitators in some training sessions have worried that the families in their communities have too many problems to take part in the program. Yet positive outcomes have been found with many kinds of families, ranging from the homeless to families whose children are actively involved in gangs, as well as middle-class families in church groups and schools. The program was developed as a universal program for all families, but most of the requests for training have come from agencies who have funds to work with at-risk populations.

Typically, the new facilitators are excited about the program and anxious to implement it with families. Occasionally there is a trainee who wants to substitute other topics for what is in the curriculum. We explain to them that the excellent research results are from groups who have implemented the program as written. If they want to experience the same positive outcomes, they must implement the program in the same manner.

Sometimes trainees question aspects of some of the content in the parent sessions, such as the use of point charts for improving behavior. We emphasize that certain trainers, as well as parents, feel more comfortable with some of the tools than others. Facilitators are encouraged to discuss and support the use of all of the tools, knowing that what works best for one family may not work as well for another.

Virginia created this program with a dream. At first, it was her hope that after the research was done, it could be used in other communities in Iowa. When it had spread successfully through the Extension system in Iowa, her goal was that it would be shared throughout the U.S. It is now in 47 states. She was amazed and thrilled to see the program endorsed by the World Health Organization (Foxcroft, 2003) and the United Nations. It has been used on five continents and in 35 countries. A dream come true, and then some.

References

Achor, S. (2011, May). *The happy secret to better work* [Video file]. Retrieved from https://www.ted.com/talks/shawn_achor_the_happy_secret_to_better_work

Foxcroft, D. R. (2003). Longer-term primary prevention for alcohol misuse in young people: A systematic review. *Addiction, 98*(4), 397–411.

Kerr, Michael E. (2000). "One family's story: A primer on Bowen theory." The Bowen Center for the Study of the Family. Retrieved from http://www.thebowencenter.org

Chapter 9

Siblings Are Special

A Practical Guide for Adapting a Universal Primary Prevention Program for Sibling Relationships

Kari-Lyn K. Sakuma, Mark E. Feinberg, Susan M. McHale, Kimberly A. Updegraff, and Adriana J. Umaña-Taylor

Starting Point

Despite the centrality of siblings in family life, sibling relationships are understudied by family scholars (McHale et al., 2012). However, sibling relationships are a rich training ground for the development of critical social, emotional, and behavioural capacities and skills that influence well-being and success throughout life. From infancy onward, sibling relationships provide a context within which problem behaviours—including aggression, delinquency, and substance use—are learned, practiced, and reinforced (Bank et al., 2004; Brook et al., 1990; Bullock & Dishion, 2002; Dirks et al., 2015; Dunn et al., 1999; Rende et al., 2005; Slomkowski et al., 2001; Solmeyer et al., 2014). Importantly, siblings and sibling relationships also have implications across a wide range of positive domains—including mental health, social-emotional competencies, academic attainment, romantic relationships, and even happiness in old age (Doughty, Lam, et al., 2015; Doughty, McHale, et al., 2015; Stormshak et al., 1996; Updegraff et al., 2002; Waldinger et al., 2007).

Sibling relationships can have significant impact on family life. The intensity and often chronic nature of sibling bickering, arguing, and fighting is reported by parents to be the most stressful dimension of family life (McHale & Crouter, 1996; Perlman & Ross, 1997) and can undermine a parent's sense of efficacy, internal resources, and competent parenting (Dishion et al., 2004; Patterson et al., 1984). Despite the implications of sibling relationships for sibling, parent, and family well-being, health, educational, social, and family services largely ignore problems in children's sibling relationships (Feinberg et al., 2012; McHale et al., 2012). Given the significant role of sibling relationships in current and future trajectories of well-being, and the potential entrenchment of sibling conflict and coercive styles, childhood is a key window for prevention strategies to support positive sibling relationships. Grounded in this literature that underscores the significance of siblings for development and well-being, the *Siblings are Special* program (*SIBS*) is a group-format program focused on promoting positive sibling relationships during elementary school via 12 weekly sibling group meetings after school and three family nights that include both siblings and parents.

SIBS: Strategy and Theory of Change

The few prior sibling interventions whose tested effects have been published generally focus on reducing sibling conflict and aggression through parental intervention (Kramer, Laurie, 2004; Siddiqui & Ross, 2004). Our *SIBS* program extended such work as a universal primary prevention program, strategically targeting elementary school-aged sibling dyads to support positive sibling relationships before the emergence of increased levels of risky behaviour commonly observed in adolescence (Feinberg, Sakuma, et al., 2013; Feinberg, Solmeyer, et al., 2013). A central feature of the program was to build warm and supportive relationships within the sibling pair. In testing the program, we found that the approach was popular with parents who were eager to find ways to reduce conflict and improve sibling relations. As the program focused on siblings and invited parents to participate in family nights to hear what their children were learning, we believed that the program would be perceived as less stigmatizing as parents might experience with a program that focused on bolstering parental deficiencies (Feinberg et al., 2012). During family nights we provided parents with approaches and support around parenting siblings—in contrast to other parenting programs focused on parenting skills for individual children. Typically, a very low proportion of eligible families enrol in multi-session parenting and family programs: In one of the most successful recruitment initiatives, high levels of resources and community effort resulted in only 17% of eligible families enrolled in a family program for sixth graders (Spoth et al., 2007). In contrast, *SIBS* recruitment rates have been several times higher than other family programs; for example, in our trial focused on Latinx families, over 80% of eligible families enrolled in the randomized trial.

The initial conceptualization of *SIBS* included a cross-cultural, multi-site plan to develop and test a program that could be applied to multiple ethnic/racial groups. Research on the sociocultural contexts of sibling relationships was being conducted by Drs. Kim Updegraff, Gene Brody, and Susan McHale, who influenced the development of the *SIBS* program. We wanted to avoid the more typical approach of developing and testing program efficacy with a single group, typically majority white, and then adapting the program for other groups as if they were variants of mainstream culture. Thus, we aimed for a diverse audience from the beginning of program development: McHale and Feinberg conducted focus groups with family members in central Pennsylvania; Updegraff conducted focus groups with Latinx families in Phoenix, Arizona; and Brody conducted focus groups with African American families in rural Georgia. Several common themes emerged across these focus

groups. Parents in both Phoenix, Arizona and rural Georgia saw sibling relationships as an important element of their children's and families' lives and
indicated that they hoped siblings would support one another, especially as
they grow older. Yet, parents also indicated that conflict and jealousy were
common aspects of family life that required parents' management. Several
similar strategies were described across the two groups of parents, including using family time as a means to promote shared sibling activities and
identifying tasks and activities (e.g., homework, chores) that siblings could
do together. Parents in both locations also noted that age and personality
differences and feelings of jealousy were significant challenges. These commonalities reinforced our approach to develop a program that was appealing
to families from European American, African American, and Latinx backgrounds. Unfortunately, NIH grant reviewers (perhaps wisely) thought that
our plan for a three-site trial was too ambitious given the program did not
have preliminary evidence of efficacy. Thus, Feinberg and McHale, who had
spearheaded the initiative, moved forward with an initial test focusing on a
sample of predominantly white families in largely rural, central Pennsylvania
with support from the National Institute on Drug Abuse (NIDA).

The development of the *SIBS* program was based on our conceptual model;
in Figure 9.1, four potential pathways are depicted through which the sibling relationship contributed to poor outcomes for children (Feinberg et al.,
2012). Path 1 represents the emergence of a generalized coercive interpersonal
style due to ongoing negative, conflictual sibling interactions (Patterson et

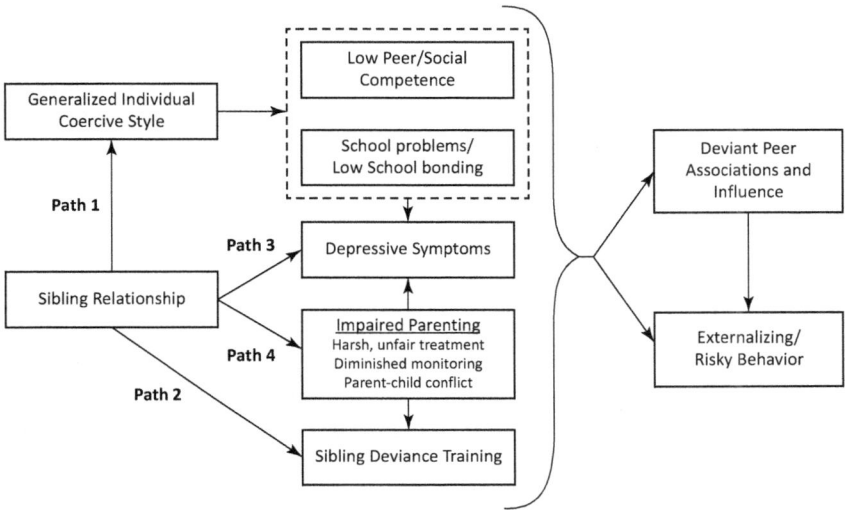

Figure 9.1 Conceptual Model of Pathways from Siblings' Relationship to Adjustment
Problem

al., 1984). In turn, a general coercive style may lead to difficulty with peers and teachers with consequences for school adjustment and performance and associations with risky peers (Dishion et al., 1991; Natsuaki et al., 2009). Through the second path, sibling relations may lead to sibling deviance training, in which siblings reinforce antisocial tendencies and may collude in opposition to parental authority (Bullock & Dishion, 2002; Snyder et al., 2005). Path 3 represents a link between sibling conflict and depressive symptoms (Gass et al., 2007; Kim et al., 2007; Milevsky & Levitt, 2005; Waldinger et al., 2007). A number of studies demonstrate a link between challenging sibling relationships and internalizing problems in children (e.g., Milevsky & Levitt, 2005). More specifically, increases in sibling conflict were linked with increases in depression over time (Kim et al., 2007). Finally, Path 4 represents the potential negative impact of frequent sibling conflict on parenting quality (Jacobson & Crockett, 2000; McHale & Crouter, 1996).

The *SIBS* program consists of 12 sessions that are delivered in 1.5-hour weekly, afterschool meetings; holding the groups after school provides children with a familiar setting for learning program content and simplifies transportation issues as both children are already at school. (See Table 9.1 for a list of session topics; Feinberg, Solmeyer, et al., 2013.) Sibling groups are generally led by two trained facilitators who work together to manage four sibling pairs. The older sibling in each dyad is in fifth grade, and the younger, in first grade or older. Each week, group leaders send home a parent letter that explains what their children learned, as well as a family activity ("fun work") to complete at home that reinforces the lessons learned during the session. At the end of sessions, group leaders are expected to very briefly check in with parents, providing them with insights on their children's interactions together and compliments on their children's learning. Three Family Fun Nights, equally spaced across the 12 afterschool sessions, also are held at school (following the afterschool session on those days); during these, the siblings' families are invited for dinner and to participate in activities. The Fun Night time is split between separate parent and child meetings and a period when the parents and children come together and children demonstrate what they have learned about how to best get along with their siblings.

Creating the *SIBS* Content

Feinberg and McHale, with the help of then-graduate students, Stephen Erath and Shawn Whiteman, along with input from Dr. Karen Bierman, created the initial session templates and activities for the sibling pilot program. Given the lack of sibling-focused prevention programming, the team was charting new territory in developing program content. Synergies with multiple areas of prevention/intervention research at the Pennsylvania State University (Penn State) contributed to the development of the *SIBS* program. Although the genesis of *SIBS* can be attributed to McHale and Feinberg's

Table 9.1 Siblings Are Special Session Description

Session #	Title	Description
Session 1	Building Positive Feelings	The session introduces the program to the participants, establishes the rules and routines of the program, fosters a positive group environment, and promotes positive sibling interaction.
Session 2	Understanding Feelings	The Traffic Light is introduced as a tool to help with self-control. Children practice identifying their own and others' feelings, and are coached in practicing to identify and express their feelings with various levels of intensity.
Session 3	OK and NOT OK	Children learn how to communicate their feelings without blaming or hurting others' feelings. They also practice hot to handle strong feelings such as jealousy and how to use the Traffic Light to calm down in stressful situations.
Session 4	Working Together	This session introduces the idea that siblings can work together as a team. Siblings will create a team mascot. Children practice listening carefully and practice self-control using the RED LIGHT to stay calm in an exciting situation.
Family Night 1	Family Night 1	Program tools and lessons are shared with parents: Red Light, Compliments, and Building a Team.
Session 5	Ears and Ideas	This session introduces the YELLOW LIGHT, in which children listen carefully to each other, discuss the problem, think of choices together, and make a plan. The focus is on generating ideas for problem solving and listening respectfully to others.
Session 6	Win-Win	This session focuses on the act of negotiating and agreeing on a good idea. Children will learn to look for WIN-WIN ideas and identify differences between WIN-WIN, WIN-LOSE, and LOSE-LOSE ideas.
Session 7	Rejection and Deals	This session helps children explore feeling rejected. They brainstorm WIN-WIN solutions to problems with feeling rejected and learn ways to be more inclusive with their sibling. They learn about how to solve problems using negotiation and that making a deal is part of being a team.
Session 8	Fair Play	This session again focuses on siblings as a team, with much time spent on ideas and practices concerning Fair Play.
Family Night 2	Family Night 2	Program tools and lessons are shared with parents: Yellow Light, Talking Stick, Fair Play, and Positive Leisure Activity Choices. Parents are also coached on how and when to intervene and help manage sibling conflict.
Session 9	Respect	The group is separated into an older sub-group and a younger sibling sub-group in order to discuss the sensitive topic of treating a sibling respectfully.
Session 10	Goal Setting	This session teaches children how to set goals specific to improving their sibling relationship. Goals setting and planning initially focuses on reducing difficulty situations. Children will then consider positive goals. This session also touches on appropriate ways to ask for help, giving and receiving social support from family members, and tattling.

(Continued)

Table 9.1 (Continued) Siblings Are Special Session Description

Session #	Title	Description
Session 11	Fairness	Children discuss perceptions of fairness in situations that involve parents' differential treatment of siblings. Children learn ways to problem solve unfair situations, and are exposed to the idea that some situations feel unfair even when differential treatment is appropriate.
Session 12	Siblings Are Special	This session focuses on the siblings' relationship and how much they have developed over the past months. The activities in this session aim to show the positive influence they have had on each other and illustrate the bonds that they have strengthened in their relationship.
Family Night 3	Family Night 3	Program tools and lessons are shared with parents: Decision-making, Respect, Fair Play, and Compliments.

prior research and discussions about sibling relationships, some of the initial operationalization of the activities and strategies was informed by the work of Penn State colleagues. For example, the original *SIBS* materials borrowed from basic peer social-emotional competence training approaches intended to reduce conflict, improve conflict resolution, and enhance positive emotional and social connection between peers in a school-setting. Most importantly, we borrowed concepts and activities from Bierman's *FastTrack* social skills training curriculum (Bierman & Greenberg, 1996), which focused on building elementary school-aged children's social skills. We also drew from the *Promoting Alternative Thinking Strategies (PATHS)* program developed by Drs. Mark Greenberg and Carol Kusché (Greenberg et al., 1995), which focused on improving elementary school-aged children's self-control, emotional understanding, and problem-solving in social interactions. The *SIBS* program adapted these programs' social and emotional skills training modules, however, to focus specifically on the sibling relationship rather than on individual child behaviour in school and peer contexts. Just as do *FastTrack* and *PATHS*, *SIBS* focused on improving children's emotional awareness, self-control, and social skills, but also included material that was specific to sibling and family relationships.

In translating the *SIBS* conceptual model to intervention activities, the curriculum team first identified as targets the qualities of sibling relationships that impacted each path. For example, with respect to Path 1, we viewed a coercive interpersonal style as leading to poor self-control, difficulty managing negative emotion, inability to communicate needs and emotions effectively, and difficulty in social problem solving (Feinberg, Sakuma, et al., 2013; Feinberg, Solmeyer, et al., 2013; Patterson et al., 1984). Thus, at the basic level, children need ways to communicate with their siblings about their feelings, and at a more advanced level, children need to be able to problem solve to reach mutually acceptable outcomes.

As the team discussed and developed activities around mechanisms for change, it was apparent that, at this age, most children need a foundation for learning and developing social and emotional competencies as precursors in order to address the higher order constructs in the model. We expected that the types of sibling relationship behaviors we aimed to promote would be dependent on each child developing increased awareness and recognition of their own emotions, capacity for behavioural self-regulation when negative emotions arise, and ability to communicate and negotiate solutions to problems with the sibling. At the same time that we aimed to develop these capacities to reduce negativity and conflict, we viewed increasing positive relationship feelings and behaviours as important for the following reasons: First, we expected that positive sibling connectedness would enhance children's motivation to reduce their aggressive and conflictual behaviours with each other. Second, we viewed a warm, supportive sibling relationship as a key influence on children's psychological well-being, and thus a counter to depressive symptoms. Finally, we expected that a capacity for empathy with the sibling's perspective and feelings of mutual support would generalize to promote children's capacity for positive peer relationships and school adjustment.

The curriculum team brainstormed activities that would support positive interactions, generate feelings of warmth, and enhance siblings' "team" identity. Thus we built in activities and messaging to convey the sense that siblings shared common ground as part of the same team; however, activities also promote children's understanding that each sibling also has special and unique characteristics to bring to the sibling team. Although content from other programs such as *Fast Track* and *PATHS* provide ideas around enhancing individual social-emotional skills and problem-solving, we worked hard to develop activities that built attitudes, skills, and understanding of one another through siblings' positive, dyadic team experiences.

An example of one of the opening activities that focuses on bringing the sibling dyad together is a discovery activity in which each sibling interviews the other about their favorite things—such as foods, games, and animals—as well as about their emotional experiences in terms of what made the other happy, mad, and proud. The program also supports siblings' positive thoughts about each other by having each child ask their sibling what they do that makes their sibling proud and what joint activity the sibling enjoys. Borrowing and adapting an exercise from Feinberg's Family Foundation program (Feinberg et al., 2009)—which he originally developed for couples based on his experience as a family art therapist—we also ask siblings to fill in a Venn diagram of two overlapping circles using art materials. Each child illustrates one part of their circle with their own, unique interests and traits, and then to fill in the overlapping area to show what the siblings have in common. As the children work on the project together, group leaders circulate to help children identify their strengths and positive attributes to include in their circle, help highlight what contributes to the siblings being similar to one another, and, as always, compliment the siblings on ways they are working well together.

Building on the Venn diagram activity, we created another activity in which the sibling dyads work to create their own team name and mascot, further building up a sense of "we" and viewing the sibling unit as a source of strength, belonging, and pride. Later in the program, the idea of a sibling team is leveraged with framing communication and problem solving strategies as ways that siblings can keep their team strong. The repetition and scaffolding of the team identity, sharing what unique strengths each child brings to their team, having the children hear repeatedly from their sibling what is special about themselves and their team, while also playing games together contributes to an overall sense of belonging to each other, developing empathy for each other, and experiencing consistent positive interactions associated with spending time with their sibling.

The next major challenge was to consider how structural elements of sibling relationships such as birth order or gender constellation may have implications for curriculum activities. First, the hierarchical nature of sibling relationships (older vs. younger, typically) means that the siblings enter the program with established power hierarchies and sibling role expectancies. Second, gender congruence may create increased emotional intensity due to both higher levels of warmth and a greater likelihood of sibling rivalry over their shared "territory" in the family.

We designed some of the activities to directly address power dynamics and strengthen positive interactions for all dyads. For example, older siblings more often serve as caregivers, teachers, and role-models; yet they can also serve as gatekeepers and instigators of risk behaviours (Rende et al., 2005; Slomkowski et al., 2001). Given their more advanced skills, older siblings also may hold greater power in choosing joint play activities, and they tend to have an advantage in games that require intellectual or physical skills. Younger siblings often complain that their older sibling has more privileges or higher status in the family, whereas older siblings often complain that the younger sibling has fewer responsibilities and is given special treatment by parents.

To address some of these structural related issues, we designed a session called "Fair Play" to introduce negotiation skills that would promote fairness, ways to treat each other with respect, and recognition of each sibling's feelings (i.e., emotion recognition and empathy). Here, the sibling dyads are split into older and younger groups to receive separate lessons using discussions and role play. The material for older siblings focuses on respecting their younger sibling and giving them chances to contribute to and direct play. Younger siblings learn what fair play is and how to be a good sport, even when a game or activity does not go as they wish. What the siblings learn during these separate sessions is then put into practice when they come together to play using what they learned about keeping their team strong through fair play.

The children first practice negotiating which game they wanted to play and then playing with a fair play approach. The game choices included in *SIBS* have a quick set up, minimal rules, and involve activities in which older siblings' more advanced skills do not yield a great advantage. Siblings practice under the supervision of group leaders who support and guide the sibling interactions while encouraging the new perspectives and skills introduced. Group leaders also compliment siblings on how they play together, and how they use the skills they just learned, and they prompt positive emotion expressions around the experience to reinforce the benefits of fair play. At the end of the session and in future sessions, the group leaders call upon this experience to remind siblings about how fun it can be to play together. In this way, the program provides layers of reinforcement for positive behaviours and warmth between siblings.

A significant family dynamic that can be related to the structure of sibling relationships is parents' differential treatment of siblings. A body of work documents that, in the face of an ethic of egalitarianism in Western societies, parents often treat their children differently, and that such differential treatment is linked to poorer sibling and parent-child relationships as well as adjustment problems in children. Importantly, however, when children understand the reasons for differential treatment and see it as fair, these negative outcomes are mitigated (McHale et al., 2005, 2012; Snyder et al., 2005). Some of our activities, therefore, were designed to address this key, sibling-related family dynamic. For example, our emotion recognition activities include a focus on feelings of jealousy, with siblings describing times when they feel jealous of one another and how they can help one another lessen these feelings. In addition, given that parents' differential allocation of privileges is a key domain of differential treatment, in one activity, children create a "family timeline" to illustrate the ages at which important milestones (later bedtimes, sleepovers) occur in their families, with discussion aimed at helping younger siblings, in particular, understand parents' reasons for their differential treatment.

Piloting

In testing *SIBS*, using internal seed grant funds, we began with two groups of four sibling dyads in a "summer camp" experience (a five-day series of morning or afternoon groups). We observed and videotaped the sessions wherein the intervention activities and modules were piloted, and our curriculum development team consulted daily, modifying activities over the course of each camp program. We received positive feedback from both siblings and parents. Siblings noted which parts of the curriculum were engaging, and parents told us that they saw improvements in sibling relationships at home during the week and shortly thereafter. We then moved to a formal pilot of the entire curriculum and procedures in a local elementary school. In this phase, we piloted school engagement, family recruitment, data collection procedures, sibling sessions, and the Family Fun Nights. This piloting was helpful in refining our procedures, the curriculum, and the evaluation measures. For example, we altered the order of sessions, moving from one that mapped onto the conceptual model of the curriculum to an order that was strategically designed to balance motivation for enhancing sibling relations with skill-building. In another step, as noted, Updegraff's team conducted focus groups with English- and Spanish-speaking Latinx families in the Phoenix area, and piloted program activities with sibling pairs during parent focus groups. These focus groups provided additional insight into the needs of parents and families generally, and feedback specific to the cultural groups involved provided a basis for a later, cultural adaptation step, as we describe later in this chapter. After a number of revised and resubmitted proposals (that most often required increased justification for our focus on siblings rather than parents), we were funded by NIDA to test the program in a randomized trial in central Pennsylvania. At the beginning of the funded project, Dr. Kari-Lyn Sakuma joined the team as curriculum specialist, having previously worked on *PATHS* adaptations and other curricula. Sakuma assisted with the redevelopment to address some of the observations from the initial pilot of the activities and to prepare the formal manualized program for implementation and initial efficacy test of the program. There were three objectives in finalizing the program for implementation: (1) reassess and modify activities for the unique sibling structure and relationship; (2) build in redundancy of the concepts being taught to the siblings; and (3) standardize the delivery of the curriculum for non-clinically trained group leaders through a manualized curriculum.

One factor we considered in revising the curriculum for program delivery was the impact of developmental differences between siblings. Although siblings' ages and developmental competencies were central in constructing the curriculum initially, we needed to modify activities further to accommodate the wide range in abilities due to the age difference between fourth and fifth grade older and second through fourth grade younger siblings (in Arizona, the program has been implemented with fifth grade older siblings and first through fourth grade younger siblings). Social skills programs are typically designed to be delivered to groups of children of similar age and ability, which means that the curriculum can be written for a certain range of language, baseline motor skills (e.g., cutting with scissors), and working memory and attention span. In finalizing *SIBS*, we re-evaluated each activity to address the wider variability in skills and development of the older and younger siblings. For example, we could only rely on very simple reading and writing skills for directions and worksheets. Although we could have relied on older siblings to explain and direct the activities of their younger siblings, we were concerned that this approach might lead to frustration among older siblings, feelings of inferiority in younger siblings, and ultimately conflict, none of which we wanted to trigger. Thus, with each activity, we replaced words with pictures for directions where possible, lowered reading and writing levels to simple sentences and fewer steps, and accompanied all assignments with spoken directions and one-on-one guidance by the group leaders, as needed.

Given the children's ages, we also minimized sitting time, and interspersed movement and activity with periods of focus that required sitting still. For example, during one role-play session, instead of handing out cards with situations written on them for sibling dyads to work through, we devised a fishing game in which siblings use a small magnetic fishing pole to catch a "fish". Siblings' jobs are to support and root for the other sibling while they are fishing. On the back of each fish are symbols that children match to a conflict scenario, and after catching their fish, the sibling pair works through that scenario together.

Another way we adjusted the curriculum to take into account the children's levels of comprehension, memory, and other abilities, was to build in redundancy in teaching concepts and competencies. Many social skills programs take this approach, such as similarly structuring all sessions. *SIBS* starts each with a welcome, moves into lessons, breaks up lessons with a snack, and provides the same closing activity so that children come to know what to expect and thereby experience a sense of mastery. Some programs also scaffold concept learning so that activities in later sessions refer back to material from prior sessions. *SIBS* was also structured in this way, and we extended this approach to teach concepts in multiple formats to increase redundancy and provide other ways for children to learn and practice concepts. We expected that short and fun lessons would also maximize children's attention and engagement.

A core component that we adapted from *PATHS* was the focus on taking deep breaths to relax and slow down reactions to maintain or regain emotional and behavioural control. *PATHS* used a traffic control signal as a tool to help students calm down when they experienced heightened emotions. We introduced this tool, referred to as a "Traffic Light" in the *SIBS* program. In initial sessions, the entire group discusses the importance of breathing, and children practice steady and slow breathing in each session. To increase active engagement and to make the experience concrete, Sakuma created the Cotton Ball Race activity—through which children learn that losing control of breathing means losing the game. For this activity, children are given a paper with a meandering path printed on it, a straw, and a cotton ball, and they are told to blow the cotton ball along the path using the straw. After the race, the group leaders lead a discussion about how hard (or easy) children found the task, and then instruct the children to try again, but this time, to blow slowly and carefully. Group leaders note children's greater success in the race on the second try and lead a discussion of why breathing slowly makes it easier to stay on the path and that when they are calm they are better able to focus; group leaders also reinforce children's fun while racing with their sibling. This activity is one that children take home as part of their "fun-work" to share with parents and as a way to connect what they are learning in *SIBS* sessions with their home environments.

An activity that builds redundancy and one that we modified specifically for promoting sibling relationships is the "Compliment Circle," adapted from *Fast Track*. We initially implemented this activity by asking the children to stand in a circle and giving each child an opportunity to say something positive about their sibling. We found, however, that many children needed additional support because they were not comfortable giving compliments to their sibling. Reasons seemed to be that family norms did not include complimenting one another; some children also seemed embarrassed about giving compliments or felt that a compliment made them vulnerable to rejection by their sibling. Accordingly, we revised the compliment circle activity using a more structured strategy. In the first session, children are asked to compliment another child in the group who was not their sibling in the context of a game. As the sessions progress, children choose who they would like to compliment, and group leaders scaffold the quality of compliments to focus on behaviours or traits rather than clothes or other superficial characteristics. Finally, toward the end of the program children are asked to specifically compliment their siblings starting with simple compliments and later, higher quality compliments, such as about their siblings' behaviours and successes during the session, or more generally on abilities or characteristics they admire. In this way, children are able to practice giving and receiving compliments and increase the power of their compliments by focusing on unique and significant characteristics and behaviours. The regular use of the compliment circle activity also made compliments a normal part of children's social exchanges, and in doing so helped to reduce embarrassment and fears of rejection. Importantly, too, each session ended with positive sibling interactions. And children enjoyed hearing the positive things their siblings and other children in the group had to say about them. One mother told us that it had been her practice to purchase a treat or prize to reward her children for good behaviour. When she offered such an opportunity to her son after he had been participating in *SIBS* however, he responded, "I don't want any THING, I just want you to say something nice about me."

Family Fun Nights are implemented for children to demonstrate to their parents the messages and tools they are learning in the afterschool sessions as well as to provide parents with information about parenting siblings—which is not the same task as parenting individual children (McHale et al., 2012). As noted, each of the three family nights includes an inexpensive dinner for the entire family and supervision and care for all other siblings. After dinner, parents and children split into two groups. One or more group leaders lead the parent group in discussions about tools and strategies they can use with siblings. Meanwhile, the children work with another group leader or leaders on a skit to demonstrate the skills and tools they have learned. Families then come together, the children perform their skits, and then families do an activity together to reinforce the lesson. Family nights end with a compliment circle—a routine that families are encouraged to engage in regularly at home such as once a week at dinner.

Results of Pilot and Efficacy Trials

The initial results from this innovative program are promising. The first randomized control trial conducted in central Pennsylvania included 174 families, and, reflecting the demographics of the region, most of the family members were white (Feinberg, Solmeyer, et al., 2013). A total of 88 families were assigned to the *SIBS* program and seemed to enjoy their participation as demonstrated through high feedback ratings and, perhaps more tellingly, their high rate of attendance. Children attended on average of 87% (10.4 of the 12) afterschool sessions and 81% of families attended at least two of the three Family Fun Nights (Feinberg, Solmeyer, et al., 2013). Results indicated that intervention parents reported less involvement in their children's arguments compared to the control group—an outcome in line with program goals given that we encourage parents to support siblings' efforts to problem solve conflicts either on their own or with neutral mediation provided by the parent (Feinberg, Solmeyer, et al., 2013). Mothers reported more fair play, and analyses of videotapes of sibling and parent-sibling interactions, rated by independent coders, revealed more sibling positivity among intervention dyads compared to control dyads who did not receive the program (Feinberg, Solmeyer, et al., 2013). We also found that children's adjustment in the intervention group was better at post-test than in the control group: We found lower levels of internalizing problems, higher levels of self-control, and higher social competence and academic performance among intervention children including as rated by teachers. Although *SIBS*'s focus is on child adjustment, mothers whose children participated in *SIBS* exhibited greater declines in depressive symptoms than those in the control group—consistent with Path 4 in our conceptual model (Feinberg, Solmeyer, et al., 2013). Taken together, the findings from the trial suggest that this sibling relationship focused prevention program, designed as a universal approach, has promise in promoting positive child and family functioning and reducing risk behaviours later in adolescence.

From this experience, we also learned that managing a group of siblings—even only four dyads—can be challenging. Group leaders found themselves managing children with high energy and strong emotions, redirecting older siblings to work with their younger siblings rather than their same-aged peers, and creatively addressing tendencies for older sibling "bossiness" and younger sibling's lower levels of attention and emotional control. We also found that the emotional intensity of sibling relations was expressed in many groups, contributing to difficulty managing sessions at times. For example, a sibling pair may come to a group session with heightened emotions lingering from an earlier conflict. Group leaders who had prior experience working with children might recognize such cues and walk the dyad through a relevant activity they had learned earlier in the program before joining the rest of the group. In other cases, behavioural challenges with a particular child meant that even two group leaders for eight children (four sibling dyads) were not enough. In these cases, an additional group leader can be provided to support that group. In supervision we work with group leaders to identify where they expected challenges in the next session, to provide ways to redirect those children during that activity, or to add some physical movement in between more sedentary activities.

Also important is that the intensity of the emotions within the sibling dyad can spill over into the emotional environment of group. For this reason, group leaders need extra support and training on managing the sibling group in ways that may be different from peer group management. In peer group contexts, group leaders may be able to use one strategy to calm the group down and bring attention back to the task. For example, when children get too silly or someone cannot sit still and begins to bother others, the group leader can choose to redirect that child to another activity or have everyone perform a breathing exercise to reinforce a skill learned earlier in the program that helps them to stop, calm down to think, and choose an appropriate behaviour. In a sibling context, not only did we need to address different levels of emotion regulation skill between age groups, but also some sibling dynamics may be so engrained that one group leader may have to lead the group while the other works exclusively with one dyad to manage disruption or help the siblings complete an activity together. In peer group settings, group leaders can sometimes rely on group norms to constrain inappropriate behaviours, such as challenging the group leader's authority, acting too silly, not following directions. In contrast, because of the familiarity and non-voluntary nature of the sibling relationship, more covert behaviours, including teasing, deliberately annoying, and partner in crime behaviours are possible.

Refining and Expanding the Program

Building on the successful efficacy trial with a predominantly European American sample our next step was to determine whether *SIBS* would promote positive relationships in children and families from a range of sociocultural backgrounds. Toward this end, we built on the sibling and family research being conducted by Drs. Kimberly Updegraff and Adriana Umaña-Taylor at Arizona State University to test the efficacy of *SIBS* in Latinx families. Initial efforts to obtain NIH funding for this project were unsuccessful given our lack of pilot data, but Umaña-Taylor secured internal funds to conduct a pilot test of SIBS with Latinx families, referred to as the *ASU SIBS Program*. Based on data from the original focus groups Dr. Updegraff had conducted with Latinx families, cultural adaptations for the *ASU SIBS* pilot study were limited to surface-structure changes (Knight et al., 2009). These changes included translating the program into Spanish, ensuring that program fliers and materials depicted Latinx families, hiring and training bilingual group leaders, and modifying examples to be relevant to Latinx families.

The *ASU SIBS Program* was delivered in five elementary schools in partnership with Arizona's largest public school district. We recruited schools where the majority of students were Latinx, ranging from 62% to 93%, given this was our target population. These schools served predominantly low-income students and all had Title 1 designations, with the percentage of students receiving free or reduced lunch ranging from 77% to 96%. Within these school contexts, it is critical to address potential barriers to program participation for low-income families. These include providing childcare to non-participating siblings who also attend the elementary school and transporting children home after the program (via a rideshare service with group leaders accompanying children to their homes). For family nights, dinner is provided for the entire family as is childcare for non-participating children and money for gas to cover transportation costs. Also like the trial in central PA, the program was offered at no cost to families and all materials were provided. In PA, siblings and families were offered $2 per session plus a $1 bonus if they attended all sessions ($25 per child total). If families were not selected for the intervention, they received the full amount for participating in the study. In contrast, the review panel for the *ASU SIBS Program* determined that families should not be paid for attendance, thus no monetary incentives were given for participation.

To test the program's efficacy, 54 families from five elementary schools were randomly assigned (within school) to either the *SIBS* program (28 families) or a no-contact control condition (26 families). Like the initial central PA efficacy trial, there was strong evidence that the program was appealing to families: 82% of eligible families enrolled in the program and 96% of those families completed the program. Siblings attended an average of 11 of the 12 afterschool sessions, and over 80% of the families attended at least two of the three family nights. Further, parents' anonymous ratings of the program were very positive, indicating high satisfaction with their program experiences (Updegraff et al., 2016).

Even with the small sample size of this pilot study, we found evidence of the program's effectiveness over the no-contact control condition, with moderate effect sizes. Findings revealed significant improvement in sibling and mother-child relationship qualities for the intervention as compared to the control condition, including in mothers' ratings of sibling relationships as more pro-social and less negative, and their ratings of their relationships with each child as warmer and less conflictual. Older siblings reported increases in emotional self-efficacy in the program group (a target of the program), and mothers reported stepping in less often to handle sibling conflicts (i.e., less authoritarian control) after the program, controlling for pre-test levels. Although parents' time commitment to the program (i.e., about six hours total as compared to 24 hours for children) was minimal, mothers in the program reported significant reductions in depressive symptoms and parenting stress compared to control group mothers. Altogether, these findings were suggestive of the program's positive impact on children's and parents' individual well-being and family dynamics via a primary focus on improving children's siblings' relationships.

With the successful pilot project and published findings (Updegraff et al., 2016), Updegraff, Umaña-Taylor, McHale, Feinberg, and Jones secured an R01 from the Eunice Kennedy Shriver National Institute of Child Health and Human Development (NICHD) to conduct the efficacy trial with Latinx families, again, in the Phoenix, AZ area. This project is currently in its second year of a three-cohort design, with a goal of studying 300 families. We are conducting a more rigorous test by comparing *SIBS* to a contact-equivalent control condition focused on academic skills and designed by our team; in the three control condition Family Fun Nights, parents receive information on supporting children's math skills, reading skills, and homework, respectively. With our larger sample size, three waves of data collection (pre-test, post-test, and one-year follow-up), and addition of daily diary data on children's sibling and family experiences, use of program targeted skills, and individual well-being, it will be possible to test mediators and moderators of program efficacy. With regard to mediators, daily diary data collected during pre- and post-test assessments will allow us to examine whether changes in program-targeted skills explain program outcomes. Further, we will test whether program effects are moderated by sociocultural strengths, such as familism values, or sociocultural risks (e.g., contextual disadvantage) to gain insights about the conditions under which *SIBS* is most effective.

Lessons Learned

A key lesson that has emerged from this line of family preventive intervention is that a focus on siblings is a game-changer in terms of recruiting families into in-person, group-format, afterschool-based sessions. The approach is not only practical—despite the need to recruit and retain multiple family members—but is a powerful means of expanding the usual scope of family programs. This success in recruitment was replicated across three projects, across two states, urban and rural schools, and two different ethnic groups.

Another lesson we learned is that a sibling focused program with minimal parent involvement can have effects on child adjustment, sibling relations, and family functioning more generally. Although we cannot disentangle the impacts of the sibling versus whole-family sessions, it is likely that these two formats were synergistic in that a modest level of parent-involvement may reinforce and thus facilitate the intervention's direct impact on siblings. Furthermore, the results of our trials with both European American and Latinx families document that the impact on the sibling relationship can be accompanied by reductions in parent depression thus supporting one of our innovative paths in our conceptual model (Feinberg, Solmeyer, et al., 2013; Updegraff et al., 2016).

Our effort to deliver *SIBS* in alternative sociocultural contexts also yielded lessons learned. Most importantly, we learned that in the face of their different circumstances—sibling relationship joys and challenges are similar such that the same kinds of skills, attitudes, and behaviors support positive sibling dynamics in both contexts. This resonated with findings from our initial focus group and piloting with Latinx families. Further, the focus on sibling relationships was similarly appealing to parents in both contexts, engendering their families' participation and engagement. An important innovation in our ongoing trial, however, will be to learn whether and how specific sociocultural factors moderate the impact of *SIBS*. Further, although the cultural adaptations we implemented were only on the surface level, we did discover different logistical considerations with these two sociocultural groups. A unique issue for Latinx families was the within family diversity of language preference— such that one parent may prefer English and the partner may prefer Spanish. This meant that additional group leaders were required so that family nights could be simultaneously led in both languages, and children's presentations would be done twice, once in Spanish and a second time in English. Further, modifications to program materials were required to provide families with side-by-side English and Spanish terminology to support within-family differences in language usage and fluency. This was important because it was also common that parents were primarily Spanish speaking while their children were predominantly English speaking. Thus, supporting a shared understanding of program concepts and terminology across languages was critical to the transfer of program learning to the family context. Finally, elementary schools that serve large Latinx student populations, and are thus most interested in collaborations, are also overwhelmingly economically disadvantaged settings (Government Accountability Office, 2016). As all partnering schools in both the pilot project and current efficacy trial with Latinx families serve low-income populations and hold a school wide Title 1 designation (i.e., 40% or more of students live in poverty; US Department of Education, 2016), addressing common barriers experienced by low-income families is critical to the successful implementation of the program in these settings.

Finally, adapting peer social emotional skill programs for the family context is a viable pathway for sibling focused intervention delivery. Sibling relationships bring strong emotional intensity to these groups making navigation of the material more challenging for group leaders as they must manage both the dyad's emotions and the impact on the greater group dynamic while delivering the lesson with fidelity. A few lessons for future studies are to provide training to the group leaders to be aware of and expect these heightened emotions among dyads, and provide extra training on how to mitigate and diffuse some of those situations. Occasionally, extra resources in the way of an additional assistant or group leader may be needed to address the needs of the individual child or group of children. Of import, this emotional intensity between siblings is precisely what brings parents in, and speaks to the salient relationship siblings hold, further demonstrating the significance of these types of family interventions.

Conclusion

In summary, our *SIBS* program has undergone a long process of development and testing. This process is not complete; instead, we view our effort as ever-evolving, with opportunities for further fine-tuning and expanding to focus on siblings of other ages, other cultural groups, and/or special populations such as families with children with special needs or chronic illnesses. Ultimately our aim is that our work contributes to an increased awareness among families, researchers, and the public, more generally, that sibling relationships can be powerful influences on lifelong health and development, that providing effective guidance for the development of healthy sibling relationships is possible, and that incorporating siblings in family research, including family focused prevention, will move the field beyond its focus on parenting of one child at a time to illuminate how families operate as socialization systems.

References

Bank, L., Burraston, B., & Snyder, J. (2004). Sibling conflict and ineffective parenting as predictors of adolescent boys' antisocial behavior and peer difficulties: Additive and interactional effects. *Journal of Research on Adolescence, 14*(1), 99–125. doi: 10.1111/j.1532-7795.2004.01401005.x

Bierman, K. L., & Greenberg, M. T. (1996). Social skills training in the Fast Track Program. In *Preventing childhood disorders, substance use, and delinquency* (pp. 65–89). Thousand Oaks, CA: Sage Publications, Inc. doi: 10.4135/9781483327679.n4

Brook, J. S., Whiteman, M., Gordon, A. S., & Brook, D. W. (1990). The role of older brothers in younger brothers' drug use viewed in the context of parent and peer influences. *The Journal of Genetic Psychology, 151*(1), 59–75. doi: 10.1080/00221325.1990.9914644

Bullock, B. M., & Dishion, T. J. (2002). Sibling collusion and problem behavior in early adolescence: Toward a process model for family mutuality. *Journal of Abnormal Child Psychology, 30*(2), 143–153. doi: 10.1023/a:1014753232153

Dirks, M. A., Persram, R., Recchia, H. E., & Howe, N. (2015). Sibling relationships as sources of risk and resilience in the development and maintenance of internalizing and externalizing problems during childhood and adolescence. *Clinical Psychology Review, 42*, 145–155. doi: 10.1016/j.cpr.2015.07.003

Dishion, T. J., Nelson, S. E., & Bullock, B. M. (2004). Premature adolescent autonomy: Parent disengagement and deviant peer process in the amplification of problem behaviour. *Journal of Adolescence, 27*(5), 515–530. doi: 10.1016/j.adolescence.2004.06.005

Dishion, T. J., Patterson, G. R., Stoolmiller, M., & Skinner, M. L. (1991). Family, school, and behavioral antecedents to early adolescent involvement with antisocial peers. *Developmental Psychology, 27*(1), 172–180. doi: 10.1037/0012-1649.27.1.172

Doughty, S. E., Lam, C. B., Stanik, C. E., & McHale, S. M. (2015). Links between sibling experiences and romantic competence from adolescence through young adulthood. *Journal of Youth and Adolescence, 44*(11), 2054–2066. doi: 10.1007/s10964-014-0177-9

Doughty, S. E., McHale, S. M., & Feinberg, M. E. (2015). Sibling experiences as predictors of romantic relationship qualities in adolescence. *Journal of Family Issues, 36*(5), 589–608. doi: 10.1177/0192513X13495397

Dunn, J., Deater-Deckard, K., Pickering, K., & Golding, J. (1999). Siblings, parents, and partners: Family relationships within a longitudinal community study. ALSPAC study team. Avon longitudinal study of pregnancy and childhood. *Journal of Child Psychology and Psychiatry, and Allied Disciplines, 40*(7), 1025–1037.

Feinberg, M. E., Kan, M. L., & Goslin, M. C. (2009). Enhancing coparenting, parenting, and child self-regulation: Effects of family foundations 1 year after birth. *Prevention Science, 10*(3), 276–285. doi: 10.1007/s11121-009-0130-4

Feinberg, M. E., Sakuma, K.-L., Hostetler, M., & McHale, S. M. (2013). Enhancing sibling relationships to prevent adolescent problem behaviors: Theory, design and feasibility of Siblings Are Special. *Evaluation and Program Planning, 36*(1), 97–106. doi: 10.1016/j.evalprogplan.2012.08.003

Feinberg, M. E., Solmeyer, A. R., Hostetler, M. L., Sakuma, K.-L., Jones, D., & McHale, S. M. (2013). Siblings are special: Initial test of a new approach for preventing youth behavior problems. *The Journal of Adolescent Health, 53*(2), 166–173. doi: 10.1016/j.jadohealth.2012.10.004

Feinberg, M. E., Solmeyer, A. R., & McHale, S. M. (2012). The Third Rail of family systems: Sibling relationships, mental and behavioral health, and preventive intervention in childhood and adolescence. *Clinical Child and Family Psychology Review, 15*(1), 43–57. doi: 10.1007/s10567-011-0104-5

Gass, K., Jenkins, J., & Dunn, J. (2007). Are sibling relationships protective? A longitudinal study. *Journal of Child Psychology and Psychiatry, and Allied Disciplines, 48*(2), 167–175. doi: 10.1111/j.1469-7610.2006.01699.x

Government Accountability Office. (2016). *K-12 education: Better use of information could help identify disparities and reduce discrimination.* Retrieved from http://www.gao.gov/assets/680/676745.pdf (pp. GAO-16–GAO-345)

Greenberg, M. T., Kusche, C. A., Cook, E. T., & Quamma, J. P. (1995). Promoting emotional competence in school-aged children: The effects of the PATHS curriculum. *Development and Psychopathology, 7*(1), 117–136. doi: 10.1017/S0954579400006374

Jacobson, K. C., & Crockett, L. J. (2000). Parental monitoring and adolescent adjustment: An ecological perspective. *Journal of Research on Adolescence, 10*(1), 65–97. doi: 10.1207/SJRA1001_4

Kim, J.-Y., McHale, S. M., Crouter, A. C., & Osgood, D. W. (2007). Longitudinal linkages between sibling relationships and adjustment from middle childhood through adolescence. *Developmental Psychology, 43*(4), 960–973. doi: 10.1037/0012-1649.43.4.960

Knight, G. P., Roosa, M. W., & Umaña-Taylor, A. J. (2009). *Studying ethnic minority and economically disadvantaged populations: Methodological challenges and best practices.* xiv, 224–xiv, 224. American Psychological Association, U.S. doi: 10.1037/11887-000

Kramer, Laurie. (2004). Experimental interventions in sibling relations. In R. D. Conger, F. O. Lorenz & K. A. S. Wickrama (Eds.), *Continuity and change in family relations: Theory, methods, and empirical findings* (pp. 345–380). Mahwah, NJ: Erlbaum.

McHale, S. M., & Crouter, A. C. (1996). The family contexts of children's sibling relationships. In G. H. Brody (Ed.), *Sibling relationships: Their causes and consequences* (pp. 173–195). Westport, CT: Ablex Publishing.

McHale, S. M., Updegraff, K. A., Shanahan, L., Crouter, A. C., & Killoren, S. E. (2005). Siblings' differential treatment in Mexican American families. *Journal of Marriage and the Family, 67*(5), 1259–1274. doi: 10.1111/j.1741-3737.2005.00215.x

McHale, S. M., Updegraff, K. A., & Whiteman, S. D. (2012). Sibling relationships and influences in childhood and adolescence. *Journal of Marriage and Family*, 74(5), 913–930. doi: 10.1111/j.1741-3737.2012.01011.x

Milevsky, A., & Levitt, M. J. (2005). Sibling support in early adolescence: Buffering and compensation across relationships. *European Journal of Developmental Psychology*, 2(3), 299–320. doi: 10.1080/17405620544000048

Natsuaki, M. N., Ge, X., Reiss, D., & Neiderhiser, J. M. (2009). Aggressive behavior between siblings and the development of externalizing problems: Evidence from a genetically sensitive study. *Developmental Psychology*, 45(4), 1009–1018. doi: 10.1037/a0015698

Patterson, G. R., Dishion, T. J., & Bank, L. (1984). Family interaction: A process model of deviancy training. *Aggressive Behavior*, 10(3), 253–267. doi: 10.1002/1098-2337(1984)10:3<253::AID-AB2480100309>3.0.CO;2-2

Perlman, M., & Ross, H. S. (1997). The benefits of parent intervention in children's disputes: An examination of concurrent changes in children's fighting styles. *Child Development*, 68(4), 690–700. doi: 10.1111/j.1467-8624.1997.tb04230.x

Rende, R., Slomkowski, C., Lloyd-Richardson, E., & Niaura, R. (2005). Sibling effects on substance use in adolescence: Social contagion and genetic relatedness. *Journal of Family Psychology*, 19(4), 611–618. doi: 10.1037/0893-3200.19.4.611

Siddiqui, A., & Ross, H. (2004). Mediation as a method of parent intervention in children's disputes. *Journal of Family Psychology*, 18(1), 147–159. doi: 10.1037/0893-3200.18.1.147

Slomkowski, C., Rende, R., Conger, K. J., Simons, R. L., & Conger, R. D. (2001). Sisters, brothers, and delinquency: Evaluating social influence during early and middle adolescence. *Child Development*, 72(1), 271–283. doi: 10.1111/1467-8624.00278

Snyder, J., Bank, L., & Burraston, B. (2005). The consequences of antisocial behavior in older male siblings for younger brothers and sisters. *Journal of Family Psychology*, 19(4), 643–653. doi: 10.1037/0893-3200.19.4.643

Solmeyer, A. R., McHale, S. M., & Crouter, A. C. (2014). Longitudinal associations between sibling relationship qualities and risky behavior across adolescence. *Developmental Psychology*, 50(2), 600–610. doi: 10.1037/a0033207

Spoth, R., Clair, S., Greenberg, M., Redmond, C., & Shin, C. (2007). Toward dissemination of evidence-based family interventions: Maintenance of community-based partnership recruitment results and associated factors. *Journal of Family Psychology*, 21(2), 137–146. doi: 10.1037/0893-3200.21.2.137

Stormshak, E. A., Bellanti, C. J., & Bierman, K. L. (1996). The quality of sibling relationships and the development of social competence and behavioral control in aggressive children. *Developmental Psychology*, 32(1), 79–89. doi: 10.1037/0012-1649.32.1.79

United States Department of Education. (2016). *Supporting School Reform by Leveraging Federal Funds in a Schoolwide program*. Retrieved from https://www2.ed.gov/policy/elsec/leg/essa/ess aswpguidance9192016.pdf

Updegraff, K. A., McHale, S. M., & Crouter, A. C. (2002). Adolescents' sibling relationship and friendship experiences: Developmental patterns and relationship linkages. *Social Development*, 11(2), 182–204. doi: 10.1111/1467-9507.00194

Updegraff, K. A., Umaña-Taylor, A. J., Rodríguez De Jesús, S. A., McHale, S. M., Feinberg, M. F., & Kuo, S. I.-C. (2016). Family-focused prevention with Latinos: What about sisters and brothers? *Journal of Family Psychology*, 30(5), 633–640. doi: 10.1037/fam0000200

Waldinger, R. J., Vaillant, G. E., & Orav, E. J. (2007). Childhood sibling relationships as a predictor of major depression in adulthood: A 30-year prospective study. *The American Journal of Psychiatry*, 164(6), 949–954. doi: 10.1176/ajp.2007.164.6.949

Chapter 10

Developing the Familias Unidas Preventive Intervention

Supporting Hispanic Adolescents through their Parents

Lourdes M. Rojas, Monica Bahamon, and Hilda Pantin

Familias Unidas

"What if we could prevent these families from needing to get to this point?" This was Dr. Hilda Pantin's thought in the early 1980s. "These families" were recent immigrants of Hispanic descent in Miami, Florida. "This point" was intensive family therapy to deal with adolescents' mental and behavioral problems, such as substance use and conduct disorders. Over the last 40 years, the answer to this question developed into what is now known as *Familias Unidas*, an evidence-based, family-centered preventive intervention that aims to prevent Hispanic adolescent behavioral problems through improving family functioning. This chapter describes the starting point and theory of change of Familias Unidas. We also discuss how the content was created, refined, and expanded throughout the years. We conclude with lessons learned.

Starting Point

As a clinical psychologist specializing in child clinical psychology and family therapy, Dr. Pantin was practicing in Miami, Florida. Miami was, and is, a hub for immigrants. A Cuban immigrant herself, Dr. Pantin's personal experience and training in Miami helped her to relate with many Hispanic immigrant families that were presenting to the Spanish Family Guidance Center, a University of Miami family therapy clinic specializing in the treatment of Hispanic adolescents with behavior problems. The stress of immigration and acculturation gaps between adolescents and parents weighed on the families. Acculturation is defined as a multidimensional construct referring to the way one adapts to the receiving culture (e.g., American) and/or retains their heritage culture (e.g., Cuban) through maintenance of values and practices (Schwartz, Unger, Zamboanga, & Szapocznik, 2010). While the adolescents were quickly adopting American cultural values and practices, the parents were less likely to do so and more likely to adhere to Hispanic cultural values. The acculturation gap between parents and adolescents exacerbated adolescent behavioral problems. The gap disrupted parent-adolescent communication and parental involvement in the adolescent's life.

For example, adolescents of immigrant parents were less likely to be deferential to parental authority, which Hispanic parents often viewed as extremely disrespectful. Parents would try to reassert control by being more authoritarian, which would then result in the adolescent seeking greater autonomy. This dynamic spiral pattern would lead to escalation in family conflict and adolescent behavior problems. Additionally, epidemiological studies paralleled Dr. Pantin's experience in the clinic. Specifically, Hispanic adolescents were experiencing high rates of substance use, conduct disorders, and risky sexual behaviors (Snyder & Sickmund, 1999; Vega & Gil, 1999), compared to their White and African American peers. Community based data portrayed Hispanic youth at the highest risk for substance use compared to their peers (Austin & Gilbert, 1989).

At the time, *treatment* of behavioral problems for Hispanic adolescents was well established, but there was not an existing evidence-based approach to *prevention* of problems among these youth. Efficacious Hispanic family therapies existed, including Brief Strategic Family Therapy (BSFT; Szapocznik & Williams, 2000) and Bi-Cultural Effectiveness Training (Szapocznik et al., 1986). However, family-based preventive interventions only existed for mainstream populations. Early work by Kumpfer, Forgatch, and Patterson (2003) suggested that parenting interventions that focused on improving family communication, parental involvement in the youth's life, and parental monitoring of youth's peer relationships could be efficacious in preventing adolescent problem behaviors. Hence, there was a need to develop an intervention that incorporated elements of evidence-based family therapy and preventive interventions, while specifically addressing the immigration and acculturation challenges facing Hispanic families.

Dr. Pantin started to brainstorm what a *preventive* intervention for Hispanic families would be. The family therapy patients that she had treated were older high school adolescents (16 to 18 year olds) with a history of years of problematic family interactions and associations with high-risk peers who exhibited substance use, conduct disorders, and/or risky sexual behaviors. By targeting middle school students, a preventive intervention would be able to enhance protective interactions in the adolescent's support systems before the adolescent was exposed to risky peer interactions in high school. Further, parents in the clinics had voiced concerns about their youth transitioning into the high school environment and experimenting with drugs and sex. This concern could be harnessed to motivate parents to develop skills to interact with their middle school adolescents that would help prevent adolescent behavioral problems in high school.

As an adolescent, Dr. Pantin had heard her parents voice similar concerns. She was often not allowed to attend social events with her friends because her parents feared the negative social consequences. With an experience herself of such parental attitudes, and the adolescent frustration and anger as a consequence, she knew that an intervention would have to do two things: there would have to be a time for adolescents to voice their opinions, but the parent had to be empowered and skilled to steer the conversation in a constructive, non-authoritarian direction.

While middle school presented an optimal point for intervention, Dr. Pantin and her colleagues also knew that intervention needed to come from a trusted source. The Center for Family Studies at the University of Miami Miller School of Medicine had a history of collaborating with the Hispanic community and Miami-Dade County public schools, and thus served as an ideal bridge to reach our target population. Furthermore, the intervention had to be delivered by people from the community that spoke Spanish and understood the immigrant experience. The team sought Spanish speaking, Hispanic immigrants with clinical backgrounds (e.g., psychologists and clinical social workers) to be the facilitators of the intervention. Our team also knew that behavior change was plausible in this population: the literature provided evidence and theory to base our intervention (Szapocznik & Williams, 2000; Szapocznik & Coatsworth, 1999).

Theory of Change

The team grounded the intervention in Ecodevelopmental Theory (Szapocznik & Coatsworth, 1999). Ecodevelopmental Theory posits that there are social interconnections between various levels of risk and protection in an adolescent's life that change across adolescent development (Szapocznik & Coatsworth, 1999). The ecological levels are drawn from Bronfenbrenner's work on the social ecology of human development: macrosystems, exosystems, mesosystems, and microsystems (1979, 1986). With the clinical experience in mind, the team conceptualized how an intervention could modify risk and protective factors at each ecological level (Pantin, Schwartz, Sullivan, Prado, & Szapocznik, 2004). At the macrosystem, we chose to reduce differential acculturation between parents and adolescents. At the exosystem, we created a network of social support for recently immigrated parents by delivering the intervention to groups of Hispanic parents and enhancing supportive connections between them. At the mesosystem, we empowered parents to develop mutually supportive relationships with school personnel and with the parents of the youth's friends to more effectively monitor the adolescent's school work and peer networks. At the microsystem, we improved family functioning through clinical strategies used in conjoint family therapy.

Creating Content

Clinical "enactment" strategies were central to content creation. Facilitators were taught how to "join" with the families, engage the adolescent, provide positive reinforcement, and redirect negative conversations. For example, if a conflict arose due to differential acculturation, the facilitator reframed the conflict by focusing on the parent's protective behaviors as an indication of their love for the adolescent, simultaneously normalizing the adolescent's autonomy seeking as part of a developmental process. Other strategies included promoting family hierarchy and increasing parental support for the adolescent.

The intervention was also grounded in participatory learning strategies (Freire, 1983). For example, in the group sessions, the parents were encouraged to share their personal experiences and how they handled difficult situations with their adolescents. The facilitator then reinforced positive behaviors and elicited parental group feedback as to why certain parental behaviors may not have resulted in the intended consequences. Since the parents were involved and engaged in the learning process, they did not feel as though they were being lectured to; rather, they functioned as the experts in developing actionable solutions for their families.

We conducted initial pilot work to test out our theorized strategies and assess the feasibility and acceptability of the intervention. Two grants, one from Substance Use and Mental Health Services Administration (SAMHSA) and one from the Department of Education allowed us to explore this work. Initially, the intervention was a multi-component, after-school program in predominantly Hispanic elementary schools delivered by study staff. The components included: parent groups to increase social support for parents, after-school tutoring to improve academic achievement, and sports programs to engage students in pro-social activities and monitor peer interactions. Qualitative feedback from the community informed us as to which components the families thought were most helpful. Specifically, they asked us to hone in on the parenting component. For example, parents reported difficulty monitoring adolescents' school engagement and peer relations because of lack of familiarity with the US school system. This difficulty stemmed from busy work schedules (i.e., a parent typically had to work two jobs to support their family), discomfort with US cultural norms, and absence of support from other parents. Similarly, school personnel reported difficulty engaging parents whom they viewed as disinterested, so we aimed to strengthen the parent/school mesosystemic component. We applied this feedback by including school counselors as co-facilitators during some of the parent group sessions. The school counselor would take the opportunity to provide support to parents, such as scheduling meetings with interested parents to discuss their concerns and link them to school resources (Coatsworth, Pantin, & Szapocznik, 2002).

Pilot work feedback also revealed that there were too many components of the intervention and it lacked structure. Since students and parents could choose to participate in any intervention component on a drop-in basis, there was not enough dosage and intensity of the intervention. The diverse, open-ended components of the intervention made it difficult to manage activities, measure progress, and engage families (who did not have the extra time to commit to all the adolescent-only activities). Furthermore, the unstructured participatory learning process, and the highly trained facilitators (Clinical Psychologists and Social Workers) needed to facilitate the intervention, did not support implementation sustainability. In these early stages, the participatory learning process involved dealing with whatever content the families chose to work on, similar to therapy sessions. In order to empower parents by deferring to their expertise and placing them in the change agent role, the team knew we had to carry forth the participatory learning strategy, yet provide more structure, dosage, and intensity. The structure also had to allow less highly trained facilitators (e.g., school counselors rather than doctoral level clinical psychologists) to implement the parent groups.

In the parent group sessions, the team established structure by using participatory learning to encourage parents to discuss the risks they anticipated their adolescent would experience during their transition to high school across the different worlds of the adolescent (i.e., family, school, and peers). They would then enumerate and explore parental protective factors in each world that could mitigate those risks. Eventually, these participatory learning discussions across numerous parent groups contributed to the material and themes that the team summarized in a structured manual. The manual outlined session topics, with talking points for facilitators, examples of parents' responses, and tips for keeping the discussion and activities on track. Dr. Pantin also started to train master level family therapists for the facilitator role, rather than PhD level clinicians, and supervise them in weekly sessions. From the weekly supervisions, we also gained feedback from the facilitators on how to address the challenges the families were facing and to develop more specific, manualized content (i.e., scripts).

In the manual, we developed scripts for the different scenarios that had been discussed in the prior group sessions. For example, a parent said they were worried about how to support their adolescents in their relationships with friends, thus we provided sample replies that the facilitator could respond with to encourage the parents to problem solve solutions. For example, "What kinds of activities can parents do with the youth and their friends so that the adolescent can spend time with friends in a safe and protected context?" Responses such as "going to the movies" or "preparing a meal together" were positively reinforced. As another example, if a parent was frustrated that their adolescent was not complying to house rules (e.g., "They never do their homework on time!"), the facilitator would allow the parents to voice concerns then steer the conversation towards skills they could use. For example, "Instead of placing the blame on the adolescent, let's try shifting the conversation. You could say 'I feel frustrated when I ask you to do your homework and I have to keep asking, what can we do differently so that you listen the first time?'" The facilitator would then have the parents practice different "I feel..." statements that correspond to the parents' concerns. The key takeaway from the content creation work and testing in the pilot work was that we needed to strengthen all the family-centered components and place parents in the change agent role for their adolescents. Thus, when we entered into the efficacy and effectiveness trials, the adolescent-only activities (e.g., after school sports) were removed from the intervention and the parent group sessions and parent-adolescent sessions ("family sessions") were more structured and guided. For the family sessions, where a facilitator would meet one-on-one with a parent and the parent's adolescent, the team followed the same topics as group sessions that had parents only. For example, if the group session was empowering the parent to practice "I feel..." statements, then the parent had the opportunity to practice these statements with their adolescent in the presence of a facilitator who would coach the parent as needed. There was also a hybrid of the family session and group session, "parent-adolescent circles", in which all of the parents in a given group would meet with their adolescents during the group to practice new interactions. The content for these circles reinforced the group and family session content; it was simply another channel to practice parenting skills.

The team also developed the sessions to go from more general parenting topics to more difficult adolescent behavior topics (such as substance use and risky sex). In this way, the family and facilitator gained each other's trust in the beginning, and, thus, were more comfortable discussing substance use and peer pressure later on. For example, towards the latter part of the intervention, facilitators would educate parents on the dangers of alcohol use in adolescence and teach them skills for how to monitor their adolescents' peers.

Refining, Expanding, Disseminating

In the first efficacy trial (Prado et al., 2007), we refined the intervention to consist of a total of 25 sessions: 15 parent-group sessions, eight family sessions, and two parent-adolescent circles. We added HIV and risky sexual behavior content because of the exacerbation of the HIV epidemic (Prado et al., 2007). The content was developed based on incorporating HIV knowledge and parent-adolescent communication about risky sex into the intervention, paralleling how we had presented communication about drugs and peer pressure. For example, similar to the substance use sessions, we first presented to the parents current statistics about HIV in South Florida and addressed common myths of HIV transmission. We then asked the parents how comfortable they would feel discussing risky sexual behaviors with their adolescent and practiced different scenarios on how and when to talk to their adolescent about risky sexual behaviors. Example scenarios included practicing how to resist peer pressure to have sex and how to practice safe sex.

Qualitative feedback revealed that the intervention was still too long, and we refined the content to further enhance a circumscribed set of the family-centered components. The focus shifted to a greater focus on parent-adolescent communication (including communication about drugs and sex), adolescent behavior management skills, and parental monitoring of peers. We dropped prior emphasis on adolescent pro-social activities because parents were very busy with multiple jobs and had limited time to engage in pro-social activities with their adolescents. Further, the parent-adolescent circles were too repetitive and lengthy. In the second efficacy trial (Pantin et al., 2003), the intervention was condensed to 23 sessions: nine parent group sessions, ten family sessions, and four booster sessions.

Once again, the length of the intervention was an issue, and parents reported some redundancy in session topics. To streamline the intervention, the manual and fidelity measures were tweaked and improved before pursuing the third efficacy trial. Manual creation was an iterative process in which clinical psychologists, social workers, epidemiologists, school personnel, and parents aided in the development. In the third efficacy trial (Prado et al., 2012), the intervention was refined to its current format—12 sessions (eight group sessions and four family sessions over three months). Not only was facilitator training more structured and centered around a more scripted manual, but the families were also provided with a parent version of the manual. Fidelity was also closely monitored by the facilitators, clinical supervisors, and adherence raters. With a random sample of recorded sessions, raters scored the facilitator's clinical skills (e.g., how well did they "join" or "engage" the family) and assessed adherence to program content. These ratings were then summarized and provided to the clinical supervisors to be able to provide feedback to the facilitators as needed. The team chose to implement this rating system, not only to assure fidelity to the program components, but also to improve the internal validity of the intervention. In other words, fidelity monitoring would assure that participants in the intervention condition were all exposed to the same intervention.

Table 10.1 summarizes each session (adapted from Estrada, et al., 2017). The intervention starts with general relationship building between the facilitator and parents, as well as general parenting skills (e.g., parent-adolescent communication). As the intervention progresses and the relationship solidifies between facilitators, parents, and adolescents, the parents enhance their parenting skills and the sessions become more focused on the more difficult topics to discuss (e.g., communication about drugs and sex).

Because of positive, repeated outcomes on family functioning, substance use, and risky sexual behavior across trials, we then conducted a real-world effectiveness trial (Estrada et al., 2017). An "efficacy trial" is typically smaller and the intervention is under a higher level of control of the researchers to ensure the program is being tested in its most robust form. In an effectiveness trial, the goal is to assess whether a program works when researchers are not as involved in the direct implementation of the intervention, but instead the intervention is managed and delivered under more realistic conditions. For example, in our efficacy trials, we had smaller samples, fewer schools involved, and facilitators who were part of the study team. In this effectiveness trial, we

Table 10.1 Familias Unidas Session Overview

Session #	Session Title	Session Content
1	Family Session #1 Engagement and Orientation	Engagement with parents and youth. Completion of family needs assessment and problem-solve family's perceived barriers to participation.
2	Parent Group Session #1 Parental Investment in Adolescent Worlds	Provides an introduction to Familias Unidas and a review of adolescent risk factors. Parents engage in an interactive exercise to discuss risks and set goals in each of the adolescent's worlds (i.e., family, school, and peer).
3	Parent Group Session #2 Enhancing Communication Skills	Focuses on the characteristics of effective family communication and parents engage in an interactive exercise to reinforce key communication skills.
4	Family Session #2 Family Communication	Parents use newly learned communication skills and practice with adolescents by discussing a relevant issue in the youth's life.
5	Parent Group Session #3 Family Support and Behavior Management	Highlights the significance of parental support, behavior management, and effective discipline. Parents complete an interactive exercise that reinforces behavior management strategies.
6	Parent Group Session #4 Parental Monitoring of the Peer World	Highlights the roles of pro-social and antisocial peers and the protective effects of parental monitoring. Parents complete an interactive exercise that reinforces parental monitoring strategies.
7	Parent Groups Session #5 Adolescent Drug Use	Focuses on the prevalence and consequences of adolescent drug use. Parents complete an interactive exercise on strategies to prevent adolescent drug use.
8	Family Session #3 Parental Monitoring of Peer World and Adolescent Drug Use	Covers family conversations about adolescent's peers. Provide ways to troubleshoot interactions between parents and the youth's peer world. Parents teach youth the skills necessary to effectively manage peer pressure to engage in drug use.
9	Parent Group Session #6 Parental Investment in Adolescent's School	Addresses the role of school in the adolescent's life and how parental connections to school can serve as a protective mechanism. Parents engage in an interactive exercise that emphasizes parental involvement in the adolescent's school world.
10	Parent Group Session #7 Adolescent Sexual Risk Behaviors	Discusses parental attitudes and beliefs regarding adolescent sexual risk behaviors, the effects of adolescent sexual risk behaviors on STIs, and what parents can do to influence adolescent behavior. Parents complete two interactive exercises to reinforce knowledge of risky sex and safe sex practices.

(Continued)

Table 10.1 (Continued) Familias Unidas Session Overview

Session #	Session Title	Session Content
11	Family Session #4 Adolescent Sexual Risk Behaviors	Parents communicate with their adolescents regarding sexual risk behaviors. Parents guide their adolescent in developing safety skills.
12	Parent Group Session #8 "Prevention Has To Be Achieved All Over Again Every Day"	Review the content of Familias Unidas. Highlight parents' role as lifetime educators of their adolescent and the importance of daily implementation of skills to improve family functioning in order to prevent drug use and sexual risk behaviors.

had a larger sample, more schools involved, and study team members trained facilitators from the schools. This effectiveness trial retained the 12-session format. Despite positive impacts demonstrated in the efficacy and effectiveness trials, Familias Unidas had some limitations regarding dissemination. The intervention was resource intensive and required compensating facilitators for many hours of work, highly trained individuals for training and supervision, and participants for transportation and their time. As such, Familias Unidas is not widely available or accessible. Thus, it was decided to adapt the sessions for online delivery.

The first online adaptation of Familias Unidas was called "eHealth Familias Unidas" (Estrada et al., 2017). The eight parent group sessions were replaced with eight videos, and the four family sessions were delivered via video-conferencing technology. The eight videos each took the form of a talk show format to provide the content from the group sessions, a portion of a culturally appropriate and engaging soap opera ("telenovela") series, and an interactive exercise. All video components were developed by the team in accordance with the Familias Unidas manual, including the telenovela series, which was developed in collaboration with a local producer and the University of Miami School of Communication. Once the parent watched the video, they then scheduled a time to meet with the facilitator through video conference. The video conference mimics the typical family session, and reinforces content from the videos. For full details on the adaptation, please see Estrada et al. (2017). All intervention content could be accessed through the eHealth Familias Unidas secure website, using a unique log-in name and password that enables facilitators to monitor session completion by the participants. Efficacy of this version has been demonstrated among parents of Hispanic adolescents in Miami public schools (Estrada et al., 2019).

In addition to increasing the accessibility and decreasing participant burden through an online format, we also had to consider the initial touch point: where could we recruit families to increase the reach of our intervention?

The first studies engaged participants through the school system and utilized school personnel as facilitators of the online intervention. There is currently an ongoing efficacy trial of eHealth Familias Unidas in primary care (Molleda et al., 2017; Prado et al., 2019) to further enhance reach. Primary care has been cited as an accessible, trustworthy source for families (Kolko and Perrin, 2014; Leslie et al., 2016; Tolan and Dodge, 2005), and qualitative feedback from our participants revealed that parents tend to trust their healthcare providers more than school personnel (Molleda et al., 2017).

We also are expanding our reach by implementing Familias Unidas outside of the South Florida area. Community organizations in Pennsylvania, Rhode Island, Arizona, and Oregon have been trained and are currently implementing Familias Unidas. Dr. Pantin and colleagues have also been involved in helping other research teams to work with Hispanic populations and incorporate elements from Familias Unidas into their interventions (e.g., an intervention that targets alcohol use prevention in Hispanic emerging adults; Petrova et al., 2019). Internationally, we have partnered with community organizations in Ecuador (Jacobs et al., 2016; Molleda et al., 2017) and Chile. In all the national and international collaborations, researchers have paid a fee to the University for our training, manual, clinical supervision, and research technology transfer.

To prepare the way for wider dissemination, a recently completed pilot trial adapted eHealth Familias Unidas to an online-only version, e-Familias Unidas, that replaced the Skype-based family sessions with online parent-adolescent interactive exercises. Parents were recruited online through Facebook ads. By recruiting participants on the most popular social media platform, providing educational videos and parent-adolescent interactive sessions online, and eliminating the facilitator component, the aforementioned participant and facilitator burdens were significantly reduced. Findings revealed the feasibility of e-Familias Unidas in retaining parents in the intervention and improving parent-adolescent communication (Rojas et al., under review).

With the latest adaptation to an online-only version of e-Familias Unidas, several questions arise for sustainability and dissemination. For example, how can we better market ourselves to communities? To date, we have been limited to grant funded projects and small contracts with community-based organizations. Similarly, how can we identify which families are most likely to engage with our intervention? We have conducted several studies to try to predict which parents are most likely to engage and attend the intervention (Prado et al., 2005; Prado et al., 2012; Rojas et al., 2020), but have not as of yet put these findings into practice.

We are also trying to understand who benefits most from the intervention. Family-based preventive intervention researchers have reported that selective or indicated interventions, compared to universal interventions, have a greater impact on family and adolescent outcomes (Sandler, Wolchik, Cruden, Mahrer, Ahn, Brincks, & Brown, 2014). Current studies are underway testing baseline-targeted moderated mediation (Howe, Beach, Brody, & Wyman, 2016). Specifically, we are testing whether the size of the benefit or impact of the program on adolescent outcomes achieved via improved family functioning differs based on baseline levels of family functioning (Rojas et al., in preparation). Findings may aid in targeting families who are most likely to benefit from the Familias Unidas interventions. Accurately screening future participants—i.e., implementing Familias Unidas as a selective or indicated intervention—may not only increase the efficiency and effectiveness of the intervention, but also allocate precious resource to those most in need.

Lessons Learned

As a team made up of professionals who were Hispanic immigrants or children of Hispanic immigrants, we were uniquely positioned to understand what our families were experiencing. We knew facilitators also had to come from a place of understanding of the unique Hispanic immigrant experience. They must be from the community and passionate about working with families. The schools, clinics, and online communities that the team utilized to reach our target populations also needed to have stakeholders (e.g., principals or physicians) who bought in to our message and allowed us to reach out to their constituencies. In other words, our consideration of community needs and our multidisciplinary team (i.e., school personnel, psychologists, epidemiologists, social workers, and public health professionals) were central to our success. For example, we built relationships with the principals in all of the schools from which we recruited families. We would invite school principals, guidance counselors, and other community advocates to our holiday parties, or we would hold a "thank you" lunch for them. Relationship building is an ongoing process, and as the team refines, expands, and disseminates our intervention, we know that these internal and external relationships need to expand and continue to evolve.

Coupled with scientific knowledge and clinical experience, our mutually supportive and trusting relationship with the community was critical in helping us come to understand what our families wanted and needed. The team also had a clear vision of what to do and how to execute the intervention. The intervention was grounded in Ecodevelopmental Theory and the literature on family therapy, family-based preventive interventions, and Hispanic adolescent development (Szapocznik & Williams, 2000; Szapocznik & Coatsworth, 1999). The team also learned the importance of manualized procedures for intervention refinement, delivery, monitoring, and fidelity. Manualization allowed facilitators to readily adhere to the intervention, and gave parents an opportunity to practice the parenting skills with their adolescents at the family sessions and later at home. As seen in this chapter, the qualitative component was integral to creating and refining the intervention content. Qualitative feedback from participants and facilitators helped in the standardization of the manual and honed the focus of the intervention. As mentioned in the previous section, more quantitative work is needed to understand who is most likely to benefit from the intervention. Researchers should carefully think through how to engage their chosen population and how to pinpoint who is most likely to benefit from which components of the intervention. Such research would assure that the team is not wasting resources or burdening participants unduly.

We also would encourage researchers to think about sustainability and cost-effectiveness from day one of intervention development. This is something the team failed to do initially, but is now actively pursuing with our online versions of the intervention. The team found that the biggest barrier to dissemination lies in accessing the resources needed to carry out the research, train, and compensate facilitators and participants. Since this was a research program, the team also did not consider how marketing could play a role in the dissemination of our intervention. The marketing of our intervention has been limited to scientific conferences and registration on lists of evidence-based programs (e.g., The National Registry of Evidence-Based Programs and Practices, Blueprints). While we now have a program website and have been attempting to reach participants via social media, we still need to incorporate evidence-based marketing strategies in future trials.

In conclusion, the development of Familias Unidas, now an evidence-based intervention, started with a question: "What if we could prevent these families from needing to get to this point?" Through clinical experience, scientific expertise, and community input, Familias Unidas was created, refined, and implemented in local, national, and international settings. The future dissemination of Familias Unidas rests in the ability of our team to evolve with technology, market to interested stakeholders, and continue to build on strong collaborations with our community.

Acknowledgements

The leadership of Dr. Guillermo Prado, Dr. Yannine Estrada, and Mrs. Maria Tapia has been central to the development and evolution of Familias Unidas. We would also like to acknowledge our research staff, students, volunteers, and Miami-Dade County Public Schools. Most importantly, we would like to acknowledge the families that have volunteered to participate in our studies.

References

Austin, G. A., & Gilbert, M. J. (1989). *Substance use among Latino youth. Prevention research update, 3*. Portland, OR: Western Center for Drug-Free Schools and Communities. Northwest Regional Educational Laboratory.

Bronfenbrenner, U. (1979). *The ecology of human development*. Cambridge, MA: Harvard University Press.

Bronfenbrenner, U. (1986). Ecology of the family as a context for human development: Research Perspectives. *Developmental Psychology, 22*(6), 723.

Coatsworth, J. D., Pantin, H., & Szapocznik, J. (2002). Familias Unidas: A family-centered ecodevelopmental intervention to reduce risk for problem behavior among Hispanic adolescents. *Clinical Child and Family Psychology Review, 5*(2), 113–132.

Estrada, Y., Lee, T. K., Huang, S., Tapia, M. I., Velázquez, M. R., Martinez, M. J., ... & Villamar, J. (2017). Parent-centered prevention of risky behaviors among Hispanic youths in Florida. *American Journal of Public Health, 107*(4), 607–613.

Estrada, Y., Lee, T. K., Wagstaff, R., Rojas, L. M., Tapia, M. I., Velázquez, M. R., ... & Prado, G. (2019). EHealth Familias Unidas: Efficacy trial of an evidence-based intervention adapted for use on the Internet with Hispanic families. *Prevention Science, 20*(1), 68–77.

Estrada, Y., Molleda, L., Murray, A., Drumhiller, K., Tapia, M., Sardinas, K., ... Cano, M. (2017). EHealth Familias Unidas: Pilot study of an internet adaptation of an evidence-based family intervention to reduce drug use and sexual risk behaviors among Hispanic adolescents. *International Journal of Environmental Research and Public Health, 14*(3), 264.

Freire, P. (1983). *Pedagogy of the oppressed* (M. B. Ramos, trans.). New York: Herder & Herder. (Original work published 1970).

Howe, G. W., Beach, S. R., Brody, G. H., & Wyman, P. A. (2016). Translating genetic research into preventive intervention: The baseline target moderated mediator design. *Frontiers in Psychology, 6*, 1911.

Jacobs, P., Estrada, Y. A., Tapia, M. I., Terán, A. M. Q., Tamayo, C. C., García, M. A., ... & Alonso, E. (2016). Familias Unidas for high risk adolescents: Study design of a cultural adaptation and randomized controlled trial of a US drug and sexual risk behavior intervention in Ecuador. *Contemporary Clinical Trials, 47*, 244–253.

Kolko, D. J., & Perrin, E. (2014). The integration of behavioral health interventions in children's health care: Services, science, and suggestions. *Journal of Clinical Child and Adolescent Psychology, 43*(2), 216–228.

Kumpfer, K. L., & Alvarado, R. (2003). Family-strengthening approaches for the prevention of youth problem behaviors. *American Psychologist, 58*(6–7), 457.

Leslie, L. K., Mehus, C. J., Hawkins, J. D., Boat, T., McCabe, M. A., Barkin, S., ... & Brown, R. (2016). Primary health care: Potential home for family-focused preventive interventions. *American Journal of Preventive Medicine, 51*(4), S106–S118.

Molleda, L., Bahamon, M., George, S. M. S., Perrino, T., Estrada, Y., Herrera, D. C., ... Prado, G. (2017). Clinic personnel, facilitator, and parent perspectives of eHealth familias unidas in primary care. *Journal of Pediatric Health Care, 31*(3), 350–361.

Molleda, L., Estrada, Y., Lee, T. K., Poma, S., Terán, A. M. Q., Tamayo, C. C., ... Prado, G. (2017). Short-term effects on family communication and adolescent conduct problems: Familias Unidas in Ecuador. *Prevention Science, 18*(7), 783–792.

Pantin, H., Coatsworth, J. D., Feaster, D. J., Newman, F. L., Briones, E., Prado, G., ... Szapocznik, J. (2003). Familias Unidas: The efficacy of an intervention to promote parental investment in Hispanic immigrant families. *Prevention Science, 4*(3), 189–201.

Pantin, H., Schwartz, S. J., Sullivan, S., Prado, G., & Szapocznik, J. (2004). Ecodevelopmental HIV prevention programs for Hispanic adolescents. *American Journal of Orthopsychiatry, 74*(4), 545–558.

Petrova, M., Martinez, C. R., Jean-Jacques, J., McClure, H. H., Pantin, H., Prado, G., & Schwartz, S. J. (2019). Mind the gap: Bridging the divide between current binge drinking prevention and the needs of Hispanic underage emerging adults. *Prevention Science, 20*, 1114–1124. https://doi.org/10.1007/s11121-019-01026-0.

Prado, G., Cordova, D., Huang, S., Estrada, Y., Rosen, A., Bacio, G. A., ... Villamar, J. (2012). The efficacy of Familias Unidas on drug and alcohol outcomes for Hispanic delinquent youth: Main effects and interaction effects by parental stress and social support. *Drug and Alcohol Dependence, 125*, S18–S25.

Prado, G., Estrada, Y., Rojas, L. M., Bahamon, M., Pantin, H., Nagarsheth, M., ... Brown, C. H. (2019). Rationale and design for eHealth Familias Unidas Primary Care: A drug use, sexual risk behavior, and STI preventive intervention for Hispanic youth in pediatric primary care clinics. *Contemporary Clinical Trials, 76*, 64–71.

Prado, G., Pantin, H., Briones, E., Schwartz, S. J., Feaster, D., Huang, S., ... Szapocznik, J. (2007). A randomized controlled trial of a parent-centered intervention in preventing substance use and HIV risk behaviors in Hispanic adolescents. *Journal of Consulting and Clinical Psychology, 75*(6), 914.

Prado, G., Pantin, H., Huang, S., Cordova, D., Tapia, M. I., Velazquez, M. R., ... Jimenez, G. L. (2012). Effects of a family intervention in reducing HIV risk behaviors among high-risk Hispanic adolescents: A randomized controlled trial. *Archives of Pediatrics and Adolescent Medicine, 166*(2), 127–133.

Prado, G., Pantin, H., Schwartz, S. J., Lupei, N. S., & Szapocznik, J. (2005). Predictors of engagement and retention into a parent-centered, ecodevelopmental HIV preventive intervention for Hispanic adolescents and their families. *Journal of Pediatric Psychology, 31*(9), 874–890.

Rojas, L. M., Bahamon, M., Lebron, C., Pardo, M., Estrada, Y., Prado, G., & Pantin, H. (under review). A feasibility trial of an online-only, family-centered preventive intervention for Hispanics: e-Familias Unidas. *Contemporary Clinical Trials.*

Rojas, L. M., Ochoa, L. G., Sánchez Ahumada, M., Quevedo, A., Muñoz, V., Condo, C., & Prado, G. (2020). Parent attendance in a family-based preventive intervention delivered in Latin America and the United States. *Health Promotion Practice,* https://doi.org/10.1177/1524839919900765.

Sandler, I., Wolchik, S. A., Cruden, G., Mahrer, N. E., Ahn, S., Brincks, A., & Brown, C. H. (2014). Overview of meta-analyses of the prevention of mental health, substance use, and conduct problems. *Annual Review of Clinical Psychology, 10*, 243–273.

Schwartz, S. J., Unger, J. B., Zamboanga, B. L., & Szapocznik, J. (2010). Rethinking the concept of acculturation: Implications for theory and research. *American Psychologist, 65*(4), 237.

Snyder, H. N., & Sickmund, M. (1999). *Juvenile offenders and victims: 1999 National Report.* Pittsburgh, PA: Office of Juvenile Justice and Delinquency Prevention.

Szapocznik, J., & Coatsworth, J. D. (1999). An ecodevelopmental framework for organizing the influences on drug abuse: A developmental model of risk and protection. In M. Glantz & C. Hartel (Eds.), *Drug abuse: Origins & interventions* (pp. 331–366). Washington, DC: American Psychological Association.

Szapocznik, J., Rio, A., Perez-Vidal, A., Kurtines, W., Hervis, O., & Santisteban, D. (1986). Bicultural Effectiveness Training (BET): An experimental test of an intervention modality for families experiencing intergenerational/intercultural conflict. *Hispanic Journal of Behavioral Sciences, 8*(4), 303–330.

Szapocznik, J., & Williams, R. A. (2000). Brief strategic family therapy: Twenty-five years of interplay among theory, research and practice in adolescent behavior problems and drug abuse. *Clinical Child and Family Psychology Review, 3*(2), 117–134.

Tolan, P. H., & Dodge, K. A. (2005). Children's mental health as a primary care and concern: A system for comprehensive support and service. *American Psychologist, 60*(6), 601.

Vega, W. A., & Gil, A. G. (1999). A model for explaining drug use behavior among Hispanic adolescents. *Drugs and Society, 14*(1–2), 57–74.

Chapter 11

Embedding a Childhood Obesity Preventive Intervention within Early Head Start Home Visits

Recipe 4 Success

Robert L. Nix

Contributors: Carrie Campbell, Pamela Cho, Sue Evans, Mark E. Feinberg, Lori A. Francis, Sukhdeep Gill, Rachel Homan, Michelle L. Hostetler, Sarah Kidder, Tiedra Marshall, Kara McFalls, Cheryl B. McNeil, Ian M. Paul, Cynthia A. Stifter, and Roberta Zelleke

---

This chapter describes the development of the Recipe 4 Success preventive intervention. Recipe 4 Success targets obesity risk in young children living in poverty through a developmentally integrated and holistic approach to behavior change. Recipe 4 Success resulted from the collaboration of university researchers and Early Head Start partners, and highlights the potential of integrating approaches stemming from prevention science and community-based participatory research.

Starting Point

Recipe 4 Success started in a barn. Each year, researchers affiliated with the Edna Bennett Pierce Prevention Research Center of Pennsylvania State University had an off-campus retreat to explore an emerging topic in the field. In 2011, that retreat was held on a farm owned by two center researchers, in their barn, and the topic was childhood obesity. The Clinical and Translational Science Institute at Penn State had identified childhood obesity as a major concern and sought to encourage community engaged research.

One colleague, Lori Francis, presented her research demonstrating the relation between self-regulation at age three, such as the ability to refrain from peaking during the gift wrap task, and trajectories of body mass index through age 12 (Francis & Susman, 2009). Another colleague, Mark E. Feinberg, made the connection between those findings and some initial conversations he and I had had about developing a new parenting intervention targeting children's emotional and behavioral self-regulation. Mark suggested we work with Lori and have the new parenting intervention on self-regulation be focused on reducing obesity risk. We approached Lori about this possibility, and she readily agreed. Soon we approached two other colleagues, Sukhdeep Gill, who specializes in community-based intervention implementation, and Cynthia Stifter, who specializes in temperament, parent-child interactions, self-regulation, and childhood obesity, to round out the core team of university researchers.

Identifying Community Partners

Early on, we decided to situate any planned preventive intervention within the context of Early Head Start. Sukhdeep had conducted a statewide assessment of Early Head Start and could identify capable and willing partners. One advantage of this approach was that Early Head Start had the same goals as we did: to improve the health and well-being of vulnerable children. A second advantage was that Early Head Start serves families in Pennsylvania who are at the highest risk of childhood obesity, namely families of color and families in rural areas living in poverty. Third, Early Head Start serves families during that sensitive period, around age two, in which taste preferences and those parts of the brain governing self-regulation are developing most rapidly. Fourth, Early Head Start already had selected and trained home visitors, and those home visitors were experienced in implementing manualized curricula. Fifth, and relatedly, Early Head Start home visitors had strong therapeutic relationships with the families on their caseloads. We would not have to invest the time necessary to recruit families and develop such relationships before testing our preventive intervention. Finally, if the preventive intervention proved to be effective, wide-scale dissemination would be easier: The national infrastructure of Early Head Start is already in place. As a result, we might be able to make Early Head Start, which demonstrates consistent but small intervention effects (Love et al., 2005), even better. The possibility of collaborating with Early Head Start was exciting from the outset.

Sukhdeep set up a conference call so that she and I could talk with directors of three Early Head Start programs and gauge interest: Ann Doerr of STEP in Williamsport, Pennsylvania; Paula Margraf of Community Services for Children in Allentown, Pennsylvania; and Kara McFalls of Community Progress Council in York, Pennsylvania. Unbeknownst to us, Ann also served on the community advisory committee of the Clinical and Translational Science Institute. It was she who suggested that the institute focus on childhood obesity as a topic in need of greater attention. Everyone recognized the prevalence of obesity among both parents and children in Early Head Start and acknowledged the inadequacy of current curricula materials on obesity. At the end of the call, all three directors were eager to create a partnership and move forward.

Understanding Context

With funding from the Clinical and Translational Science Institute, we organized two full-day meetings to bring together university researchers and Early

Head Start administrators, clinical supervisors, nutrition educators, and home visitors. Before defining an intervention strategy, we needed to learn more about the specific experiences and challenges faced by the families we would be working with. We also needed to learn what was and was not feasible in the context of Early Head Start home visits, so we could embed our intervention more seamlessly within them.

In these meetings, the Early Head Start partners shared their first-hand knowledge of the ecology of childhood obesity and food insecurity among families in poverty. They highlighted many issues that have been featured widely in prior research (Paxson, Donahue, Orleans, & Grisso, 2006), as well as how those issues played out in their local communities. For example, the Early Head Start partners described food deserts, noting that many families purchase much of their food at large gas station convenience stores, the rural equivalent of an urban bodega. The Early Head Start partners talked about how high-quality nutritious food was expensive and did not taste as good as some of the fast food alternatives.

Early Head Start partners also identified issues that had not received as much attention in empirical research. For example, sometimes Early Head Start home visitors took families to local farmers' markets, but the parents were unfamiliar with much of the produce that was for sale and could not prepare it. Early Head Start partners noted that many parents have limited cooking skills in general. Many parents are young and still have the palate and taste preferences of teenagers. Even when parents have access to more nutritious food, they often do not like it and are disinclined to choose it for their families.

The Early Head Start partners described how difficult it can be to discuss food. If parents themselves have poor diets, it is challenging to talk about the importance of feeding children more nutritious food without coming across as judgmental. These dynamics are even more delicate around childhood obesity, especially if parents are overweight. Home visitors stated they never use the words "childhood obesity" with parents, but rather rely on the positive reframe, "healthy eating habits." Sometimes home visitors are in the uncomfortable position of contradicting the advice of extended family members and neighbors who tell parents their normal-weight children are too thin and need to be eating more.

Intervention Strategy and Theory of Change

From the beginning, our vaguely articulated intervention strategy and theory of change involved helping parents to promote children's self-regulation as a means of reducing obesity risk. We were aware of research showing it was not caregiving behaviors, in general, but rather scaffolding, in particular, that is most highly related to children's self-regulation (Hughes & Ensor, 2009; Hustedt & Raver, 2002; Pratt, Kerig, Cowan, & Cowan, 1988). We broadly conceived of scaffolding as the ability to structure tasks and titrate support to ensure child success with maximum autonomy. We broadly conceived of self-regulation as the ability to manage actions and responses in pursuit of a goal (Jahromi & Stifter, 2008). Self-regulation includes the inter-related abilities to direct and sustain attention, inhibit impulses, plan and sequence actions, execute flexible problem solving strategies, tolerate frustration, monitor progress toward a goal, and make necessary corrections (Bauer & Baumeister, 2011; Karoly, 1993). Although mechanisms linking self-regulation and childhood obesity are not fully specified, self-regulation might enhance agency and thereby reduce perceived stress, as well as the cravings for carbohydrates and storage of fat that result from that stress (Moore & Cunningham, 2012).

During that first meeting with our Early Head Start partners, we shared what we knew about self-regulation and childhood obesity. Cindy talked about how self-regulation is a super-ordinate construct that helps organize and explain much of child development during the toddler period, including the precursors to childhood obesity. Lori discussed research findings about responsive feeding practices that support self-regulation, such as letting children serve foods for themselves and respecting children's assertions of being full without pressuring the children to eat more.

Early Head Start partners appreciated the importance of self-regulation but did not have any systematic strategies to promote it. They believed that a focus on self-regulation would be appealing to the parents they work with. According to our Early Head Start partners, few parents think about childhood obesity or consider it an important issue. The reason most parents enroll in Early Head Start and participate in the weekly home visits is because they want their children to be well-behaved and do well in school. To be more aligned with parents' concerns, we realized we needed to tone down the focus on childhood obesity as the ultimate outcome of our preventive intervention and concentrate more on how self-regulation is related to a wide range of important outcomes.

Creating Content: Information and Learning Activities

During the second all-day meeting with our Early Head Start partners, we identified the kinds of messages about responsive feeding practices we wanted to emphasize. We also brainstormed different activities that might help scaffold the development of self-regulation. Mark described how parents could promote such skills through the simplest of everyday activities, like rolling a ball back and forth, by helping children slow down and pay careful attention to what they are doing.

First Draft of the Curriculum

In the first draft of the curriculum, there were 13 lessons, three of which were composed by Early Head Start partners from each of the centers. Each lesson contained some information about self-regulation or healthy eating habits, which required about 15 minutes to cover, and one child-friendly activity, which required about 10 minutes.

The curriculum began by defining self-regulation, in plain language, and explaining how it was critical to good behavior, doing well in school, and healthy eating habits. The curriculum noted how self-regulation operated at both psychological and physiological levels. Parents could support self-regulation at the psychological level by helping their children do things like take turns. Parents could support self-regulation at the physiological level by ensuring that children got enough high-quality sleep, maintained a consistent routine across days, and ate nutritious foods. There was some information on the biological mechanisms linking sleep quality and weight gain. There was a simple diagram showing how blood glucose levels and energy fluctuates across the day. There was some information on the importance of eating regular meals and snacks, including a summary of research on the relation between eating breakfast and receiving better grades in school. Parents would learn about appropriate portion size and strategies to encourage fruit and vegetable consumption, such as letting children choose among healthy options and using healthy dips. The curriculum noted that children, like adults, feel stress and identified ways to reduce that stress. Reinforcing Early Head Start messages, the curriculum emphasized the importance of language development so children could communicate what they needed. Finally, there was some information on the effects of media on children and the importance of being intentional in its use.

The activities in that first draft of the curriculum included learning a song written by one Early Head Start partner, Roberta Zelleke, to help children distract themselves when having to wait. One activity had parents and children work together to build a block tower. Another activity had them dance to music then freeze when the music paused. We planned to have parents create daily routine picture books, including bedtime rituals. Parents would watch a video demonstrating ways to talk to children about emotions. Parents and children also would make finger puppets depicting different feelings. We would have home visitors show parents how to read to their children in an interactive manner and give the families a silly book about fruits and vegetables to keep for themselves. Finally, for four lessons, parents and children would make simple recipes, such as trail mix or cheese quesadillas, with ingredients provided by us.

Focus Groups with Home Visitors and Parents

Once the first draft of the curriculum was completed, we conducted separate focus groups with home visitors and with parents at each of the three Early Head Start centers. Virtually all of the home visitors were enthusiastic about the prospect of the new preventive intervention. They believed that many of their families would benefit from it. The home visitors appreciated the ways in which the curriculum wove together several disparate but familiar messages they tried to convey in the course of their work. The home visitors did not anticipate challenges to completing any of the curriculum activities.

Like the home visitors, the parents also showed interest in the new preventive intervention. Parents recognized the importance of self-regulation, and agreed that helping children learn to like healthy foods was an important goal. None of the parents objected to the content of the curriculum or had recommendations for major revisions.

Despite that positive feedback, we started to get nervous. Some parents in the focus groups talked a lot and already seemed to know quite a bit about self-regulation and healthy eating habits. However, by the way some of them described interacting with their children, we wondered whether they might be too directive to optimally scaffold children's learning. Some other parents were very quiet. We wondered whether we were explaining everything to them in accessible terms, and we could not tell how engaged they might be with their children. We worried the curriculum might not be different enough from standard Early Head Start lessons to help the parents we met learn new ways of interacting with and supporting their children.

New Direction for the Curriculum

On the drive home from the final focus groups, Lori and I discussed revamping the curriculum to better meet the needs of more families. The new curriculum needed to focus less on imparting new information and more on helping parents be actively involved in learning new skills. The curriculum needed to be standardized, as it had always been, but it also needed to be more adaptable to better accommodate the wide range of families in Early Head Start.

On that drive, we considered the possibility of using food preparation activities as the focus of each lesson. I recalled making cookies once with two young children who were so excited they struggled to control themselves. This seemed like an ideal state in which to learn self-regulation. I also recalled a conversation I had with Cheryl McNeil several years earlier. She observed that, when parents become proficient in parent-child interaction therapy techniques, such as behavior descriptions (McNeil & Hembree-Kigin, 2010), children often exhibit more elaborated play, longer bouts of sustained concentration, and greater persistence in the face of obstacles. We had included recipes in some lessons to provide families with healthy snack and meal options but that was all. We now recognized the opportunity to use food preparation activities as the focus of each lesson and use parent-child interaction therapy techniques as a means of structuring those activities. We could simplify the information content we had developed and use it as a framing mechanism to emphasize the many ways in which self-regulation applies to daily activities, including cooking.

In this new approach, home visitors would not interact directly with the children, but rather stand back and coach the parents as they complete the food preparation activities with the children. This would compel all parents to be more engaged. One of the unique strengths of parent-child interaction therapy is that it assumes a behavioral approach to teaching parents to be engaged—without taking over—in ways children perceive as highly reinforcing, validating, and responsive. For our preventive intervention, we decided to focus on three core parenting behaviors: (1) describing what children are doing as a means of showing interest and helping them focus and sustain concentration; (2) offering meaningful choices to enhance self-efficacy and increase investment in the final snack or meal; and (3) praising effort. These three behaviors might be easier for parents to learn, apply, and generalize than higher-level principles about sensitively scaffolding children's self-regulation, yet accomplish similar ultimate goals.

There are distinct benefits in using food preparation activities to teach parents to sensitively scaffold children's self-regulation. Few parents have tried to cook with such young children before. We can honestly tell parents that these activities are hard for all children, but that parents can make the activities successful by engaging in the three core parenting behaviors. We think it is easier to teach parents the three behaviors in a new activity, rather than trying to get them to change something they already are doing with their children.

Compared to anything else we could think of, food preparation activities provide more opportunities for parents to hone their abilities to scaffold and for children to practice self-regulation. Food preparation activities can help children learn to focus and concentrate over extended periods of time. The activities help children learn to control their bodies, as they do something like stirring ingredients together without spilling. The activities also help children learn to wait and link current actions with future rewards, as they anticipate eating a special frozen dessert. While parents and children are making each snack or meal, home visitors can point out the different opportunities to count or identify colors and textures. Home visitors can have parents and children take turns while adding successive ingredients to something like a yogurt parfait. In addition, home visitors can maximize occasions for parents and children to coordinate their actions and work toward a common goal, such as having parents hold grapes steady while children slice them in quarters with a plastic knife. We believed there would be great value in having parents and children repeatedly participate in activities that require extended periods of joint attention to complete multiple sequential steps in a process. We believed children would be especially eager to practice self-regulation because of their natural motivation to be involved in meaningful adult activities (Rheingold, 1982; Svetlova, Nichols, & Brownell, 2010).

Food preparation activities provide many occasions in which home visitors can casually introduce bits of information about responsive feeding practices and healthy eating habits in the context in which the information is relevant, without seeming overly pedantic. Food preparation activities also provide many occasions to introduce children to new healthy foods. We know children are more likely to eat foods they help prepare (Knai, Pomerleau, Lock, & McKee, 2006).

We hoped the recent surge in the popularity of cooking shows might inspire parents to want to cook more. If the lessons are successful and parents and children enjoy cooking together, parents might be more likely to sustain the practice. Importantly, we are not asking parents to add something new to their schedules, such as special child play time, which is standard in parent-child interaction therapy. Rather we are just asking them to take a little more time and include their children in something they already have to do. Across the world, preparing food is a part of holidays and celebrations. Cooking and feeding are a fundamental way in which we take care of one another and communicate feelings of appreciation and love. We hoped we could tap into those primal instincts and help parents feel even more connected to and competent in their caregiving role.

We decided the second draft of the curriculum should be a little shorter. Each of the 10 lessons includes a detailed outline as well as a verbatim sample script that identifies multiple opportunities in which home visitors can encourage parents' use of descriptions, giving choices, and praise for effort. Each lesson includes a little information about self-regulation skills or healthy eating habits prior to and after the food preparation activity. Each lesson structures the sharing of the snack or meal so that parents and home visitors can model enjoyment of healthy eating, and children can receive more praise for their work. We include a brief mindfulness activity before eating and explain to parents how sitting together at the table and focusing on what we are eating is beneficial to everyone. We have parents identify ways in which they can generalize new principles throughout the week and post those ideas on the refrigerator with special fruit and vegetable magnets. Each week we have parents add the new recipe to a recipe book we supply at the beginning of the intervention, and we leave extra ingredients with families so they can re-make the snacks and meals on their own. Both home visitors and parents complete short surveys at the end of each lesson. Items on the surveys ask how much parents have described behavior, given choices, and praised effort. In addition to assessing implementation quality, we want to use the surveys to remind home visitors and parents of the importance of the core behaviors to scaffolding children's self-regulation.

Refining and Expanding the Preventive Intervention

After implementing the first randomized controlled trial of Recipe 4 Success (Nix et al., in press), we decided to make four substantive changes to the curriculum before conducting the second trial. First, Cheryl convinced us to add reflections as a fourth core parenting behavior. In our case, reflections are defined as repeating back what children say before expanding on those utterances or answering questions. Borrowed from speech therapy, this skill should help to further improve child language, a strong predictor of self-regulation (Vallotton & Ayoub, 2011). Moreover, it is one additional way in which parents can show children they are paying close attention to what the children are doing.

Second, we were worried that it was too hard for home visitors to teach the four core parenting behaviors and introduce parents to the food preparation activities simultaneously. Thus, we decided to add two lessons in which we just focus on teaching the four core parenting behaviors. Home visitors define and demonstrate a behavior and then have parents practice it. Once parents become proficient at each behavior, home visitors have parents practice using all behaviors at the same time.

Third, in the first trial, we learned that many families did not have kitchen essentials, such as a microwave-safe bowl or measuring cups and spoons. Thus, we now supply each family with these items, which we give out across several of the early lessons. We hope these small gifts help generate positive regard for Recipe 4 Success and help make up for the discomfort some parents feel at having to learn so many new behaviors in short succession.

Finally, we decided to swap out several of our recipes to make them even more healthy. We especially liked the prospect of being able to help parents learn to cook with their Special Supplemental Nutrition Program for Women, Infants, and Children (WIC) ingredients as one additional benefit of Recipe 4 Success. As a result, our new criteria for all recipes is that they consist of three to five WIC ingredients (and nothing else), at least one fruit or vegetable, and a source of protein, if possible. The recipes can take no more than a few minutes to prepare and require nothing more than a microwave or freezer. We include a wide variety of novel and familiar ingredients and include some recipes appropriate for breakfast, lunch, dinner, and dessert.[1] In addition to the recipes we feature in the lessons, we also send out additional sets of three or four recipes as boosters three and nine months after Recipe 4 Success is over, with reminders for parents to use the four core parenting behaviors while preparing the recipes with their children.

Lessons Learned

The two biggest challenges for Recipe 4 Success involve implementation fidelity and Early Head Start center capacity. Because Recipe 4 Success is designed for children, age two, only a small percentage of Early Head Start families participate in the program at any one time. This makes it challenging to discern the optimal approach to implementation support. Early Head Start supervisors are reluctant to devote too much time of their group or individual supervision time to Recipe 4 Success because other families on the home visitors' caseloads need attention too. In the second trial of the preventive intervention, we had home visitors audio record three of their lessons. We hoped to be able to provide some feedback to the home visitors on a timely basis, but that proved impossible. Home visitors sometimes failed to send us the recordings promptly, and it took us a long time to listen to the recordings and write comments. Moreover, for understandable reasons, Early Head Start supervisors wanted to be able to approve what we shared with home visitors, so that our comments were consistent with broader goals in supervision. In future trials, it would be helpful to work more intensively with the supervisors themselves so they are in a better place to support implementation fidelity. Perhaps, the supervisors could be involved in leading the home visitor training to further ensure their own mastery of content, and the supervisors and home visitors could listen to parts of audio recordings together. The supervisors need to be as well-versed and invested in the goals of Recipe 4 Success as the study investigators.

The other challenge for Recipe 4 Success involved Early Head Start center capacity for implementation. Across the first trial, which involved three Early Head Start centers, and the second trial, which involved those three centers plus four more, every Early Head Start center we approached was eager to partner with us. We discussed with administrators what the basic consultation model would be: One designated time each week in which all home visitors delivering the program would be available for a 30-minute conference call to report progress, ask questions, and receive suggestions for overcoming obstacles. All Early Head Start programs were willing to make this commitment. However, some Early Head Start programs were willing to make this conference call part of the pre-existing and regularly scheduled group supervision, and some Early Head Start programs made this conference call a new commitment for Early Head Start home visitors. Although not always the case, this latter model of consultation was more prone to problems. Home visitors often called in from different locations, so the shared experience of implementing the program was not as apparent. Some home visitors regularly had other issues that prevented their being able to call in. And, without a supervisor always present, it was difficult for us to instill the message that these conference calls were imperative for implementation fidelity and critical to success. In the future, we most likely would require that conference calls be part of the standing group supervision that all Early Head Start programs already have in place.

Concluding Remarks

Recipe 4 Success focuses on ways to improve parents' sensitive scaffolding as a means of enhancing children's self-regulation and reducing obesity risk. We are ambitious in the amount of material we present across the curriculum, but we try to make all of that material less overwhelming by tying everything together with overarching conceptual themes related to self-regulation. Importantly, we try to frame everything we do according to the parents' identified goal of having children who are well-behaved and do well in school.

Recipe 4 Success relies on some of the active coaching techniques developed in parent-child interaction to teach parents concrete ways to sensitively scaffold children's self-regulation. By making these techniques an integral part of the curriculum and explicit to the parents, we hope it is easier for home visitors to provide multiple gentle reminders and feedback as necessary until parents are competent at the new behaviors. We chose to rely on food preparation activities every week to ensure that parents and children are engaged rather than passively receiving information they might apply in the future. These food preparation activities, made with ingredients provided by us, help parents see that their children will eat more healthy foods than expected, and the activities help parents see how eager children are to help out. By the end of the preventive intervention, parents have a colorful recipe book with almost 20 recipes that require only WIC ingredients. We hope parents use these recipes as a new way to spend meaningful quality time with their children.

We have no doubt that our willingness to completely revamp the first version of the curriculum and change the focus of the learning activities improved the potential impact of Recipe 4 Success. The tightly-sequenced and highly-structured food preparation activities make the current lessons unique from standard Early Head Start home visits.

The development of Recipe 4 Success reflected the accumulated wisdom of multiple university researchers and Early Head Start partners, all of whom had been working to help families in multiple community-based preventive interventions and human service organizations for many years. As such, Recipe 4 Success capitalizes on the particular strengths and insights of both prevention science and community-based participatory research in an innovative approach to reducing obesity risk among young children living in poverty.

Acknowledgements

The development of the Recipe 4 Success preventive intervention relied on the efforts of a large team of university researches and community-based partners. We are grateful to all the Early Head Start home visitors and parents who have worked with us over the last seven years and provided feedback about ways to improve our preventive intervention. The development of Recipe 4 Success was funded by the National Center for Advancing Translational Sciences (grant UL Tr000127 to the Clinical and Translational Science Institute of Pennsylvania State University), the Eunice Kennedy Shriver National Institute of Child Health and Human Development (grant R01HD081361), and the Social Sciences Research Institute and Edna Bennett Pierce Prevention Research Center of Pennsylvania State University. Correspondence about this chapter should be sent to Robert Nix at robert.nix@wisc.edu.

Note

1   In the future, we might continue to refine the recipes. We tried to make the recipes interesting and somewhat challenging. However, we failed to appreciate the common reluc-

tance of toddlers to eat foods with multiple ingredients mixed together. Numerous times home visitors have reported that children will eat each ingredient separately as they are preparing the recipes but will not eat the final meal or snack. It might be better to have more recipes in which ingredients are indistinguishable from one another or completely separate.

References

Bauer, I. M., & Baumeister, R. F. (2011). Self-regulatory strength. In K. D. Vohs & R. F. Baumeister (Eds.), *Handbook of self-regulation: Research, theory, and application* (2nd ed.) (pp. 64–82). New York: Guilford Press.

Francis, L. A., & Susman, E. J. (2009). Self regulation and rapid weight gain in children from age 3 to 12 years. *Archives of Pediatrics and Adolescent Medicine, 163*(4), 297–302.

Hughes, C. H., & Ensor, R. A. (2009). How do families help or hinder the emergence of early executive function? *New Directions for Child and Adolescent Development, 123*(123), 35–50.

Hustedt, J. T., & Raver, C. C. (2002). Scaffolding in low-income mother-child dyads: Relations with joint attention and dyadic reciprocity. *International Journal of Behavioral Development, 26*(2), 113–119.

Jahromi, L. B., & Stifter, C. A. (2008). Individual differences in preschoolers' self-regulation and theory of mind. *Merrill-Palmer Quarterly, 54*(1), 125–150.

Karoly, P. (1993). Mechanisms of self-regulation: A systems view. *Annual Review of Psychology, 44*(1), 23–52.

Knai, C., Pomerleau, J., Lock, K., & McKee, M. (2006). Getting children to eat more fruit and vegetables: A systematic review. *Preventive Medicine, 42*(2), 85–95.

Love, J. M., Kisker, E. E., Ross, C., Raikes, H., Constantine, J., Boller, K., … Vogel, C. (2005). The effectiveness of early head start for 3-year-old children and their parents: Lessons for policy and programs. *Developmental Psychology, 41*(6), 885–901.

McNeil, C. B., & Hembree-Kigin, T. L. (2010). *Parent-child interaction therapy* (2nd ed.). New York: Springer.

Moore, C. J., & Cunningham, S. A. (2012). Social position, psychological stress, and obesity: A systematic review. *Journal of the Academy of Nutrition and Dietetics, 112*(4), 518–526.

Nix, R. L., Francis, L. A., Feinberg, M. E., Gill, S., Jones, D. E., Hostetler, M. L., & Stifter, C. A. (in press). Improving toddlers' healthy eating habits and self-regulation: A randomized controlled trial. *Pediatrics.*

Paxson, C., Donahue, E., Orleans, C. T., & Grisso, J. A. (Eds.). (2006). Childhood obesity (Special Issue). *The Future of Children, 16.*

Pratt, M. W., Kerig, P., Cowan, P. A., & Cowan, C. P. (1988). Mothers and fathers teaching 3-year-olds: Authoritative parenting and adult scaffolding of young children's learning. *Developmental Psychology, 24*(6), 832–839.

Rheingold, H. L. (1982). Little children's participation in the work of adults, a nascent prosocial behavior. *Child Development, 53*(1), 114–124.

Svetlova, M., Nichols, S. R., & Brownell, C. A. (2010). Toddler's prosocial behavior: From instrumental to empathic to altruistic helping. *Child Development, 81*(6), 1814–1827.

Vallotton, C., & Ayoub, C. (2011). Use your words: The role of language in the development of toddlers' self-regulation. *Early Childhood Research Quarterly, 26*(2), 169–181.

Part IV

Family Transitions

Chapter 12

Developing the Nurse-Family Partnership

David Olds and Elly Yost

Starting Point

Nurse-Family Partnership (NFP) is a program of prenatal and infancy/toddler home-visiting by registered nurses for low-income mothers with no previous live births. NFP nurses work with mothers, fathers, and other caregivers to address three overarching goals: (1) to improve pregnancy outcomes by promoting women's prenatal health; (2) to improve children's health and development by promoting parents' competent care of their children; and (3) to enhance parents' health and life-course by guiding women to reduce closely spaced subsequent pregnancies, complete their educations, and find work to sustain their family. Nurses link families with needed services and, when possible, involve other family members (especially children's fathers and grandmothers) in the visits. Program practices, as discussed below, are grounded in developmental epidemiology and theories of human-attachment (Bowlby, 1969), human-ecology (Bronfenbrenner, 1979), and self-efficacy (Bandura, 1977).

Today, the program is operating in 41 states in the US, the US Virgin Islands, five US Tribal Nations, and seven other countries, including England, Scotland, Northern Ireland, Norway, Bulgaria, Canada, and Australia, where it is offered exclusively to Aboriginal and Torres Strait Islander families. It is available in every community in mainland Scotland. NFP is adapted to individual needs and cultures while ensuring that it is conducted in alignment with its essential model elements that characterize the program tested in a series of randomized clinical trials conducted over the past four decades.

The program can be traced to David Olds's experience working in an inner-city daycare center in 1970 and 71, where he witnessed the aftermath of children's prenatal exposure to drugs and alcohol and child maltreatment. As a result of these observations, he created a parent-group meeting in the center held while children napped, but it was the parents of children he was least concerned about who showed up for the meetings. While this may have been a reflection of some parents working during the hours when the center was open, those he wanted most to engage did not respond to his efforts to communicate with them. This experience led him to conclude that for many children in his preschool classroom, it was already too little and too late. These experiences led him to become interested in improving prenatal influences on health and development along with promoting parents' abilities to accurately read and respond to young children's communicative signaling as a foundation for building a sense of security on the part of the child, preventing child abuse and neglect, and promoting children's language and cognitive development. Given that many adversities that compromise parents' care of themselves and their children were traced epidemiologically to conditions in the home and neighborhood, David decided to focus on low-income parents, supporting care of their children in their homes.

As an undergraduate at Johns Hopkins, David had studied and worked with Mary Ainsworth (Ainsworth et al., 1978), a professor of developmental psychology who was centrally involved in developing the evidentiary foundations for John Bowlby's attachment theory (Bowlby, 1969). This experience led David to develop a deep commitment to helping parents provide competent care for their children, building upon their evolutionary-grounded instinct to protect their offspring (Swain et al., 2014). Observing the inner-city environment in which families lived, however, drew his attention to those social and material contexts that limited parents' abilities to protect themselves and their children. After working for two years in this setting, he went to graduate school at Cornell to work with Urie Bronfenbrenner, widely considered the father of human ecology theory (Bronfenbrenner, 1979). It was at Cornell that David developed his commitment to testing interventions in randomized trials to determine whether they deserved public policy support. He developed the original proposal for the NFP while finishing his dissertation at Cornell and working in a non-profit agency in Elmira, NY that received the federal Maternal and Child Health research grant to conduct the first NFP trial.

Not knowing a thing about obstetrics or pediatrics, he developed a relationship with co-investigators Dr. Robert Tatelbaum (an obstetrician) and Dr. Robert Chamberlin (a pediatrician) from the University of Rochester. They were centrally involved in deepening the underlying health content of the program. Whatever David has come to know about nursing can be traced to his good fortune of having worked with incredibly passionate, insightful, and smart nurses, starting in 1977 with his daily collaboration with the Elmira team of nurse home visitors: Georgie McGrady, Diane Farr, Liz Chilson, Lynn Scazafabo, and Jackie Roberts.

The commitment to strong evidence along with deep attention to program design (discussed below) help account for NFP's having been identified, so far, as the only prenatal or early childhood program that meets the "Top Tier" of evidence established by the nonprofit philanthropy Evidence-Based Programs (Social Programs That Work, 2020, https://evidencebased-programs.org/).

Strategy and Theory of Change

Research-Based

The program has been grounded in an understanding of what segments of the population are at greater risk for poor pregnancy outcomes, compromised child health and development, and diminished economic self-sufficiency on the part of parents, and at what point in human development we have the greatest opportunity to improve maternal and child health. Reviews of this literature led to a focus on women who were bearing their first children and who were either poor, unmarried, or teenaged, given that women with these characteristics generally are at greater risk for poor maternal and child outcomes.

In addition, starting with the Elmira trial, we reviewed the epidemiological literature to identify modifiable factors that predict pregnancy outcomes, child health and development, and maternal life-course. These factors became the targets for behavioral change during pregnancy and the early years of the first child's life, and served as the foundation for NFP program content. We continue to review this literature to ensure that program content aligns with state-of-the-art evidence on predictors of maternal and child health during pregnancy and the first two years of life.

Theoretical Foundations

The program has been guided by three fundamental theories that help organize influences on parents and children early in life into a coherent framework designed to facilitate nurses' support of parents' adaptive behavioral change. The first, noted above, is attachment theory. This theory emphasizes that responsive early parental caregiving attuned to infants' communicative signaling creates a sense of trust on the part of young children that allows them to explore the world with confidence (Bowlby, 1969; Ainsworth et al., 1978). And, evidence is accumulating that human caregivers, in spite of individual experiences and cultural influences on their parenting behaviors, are instinctually driven to protect their offspring (Swain et al., 2014; van't Veer et al., 2019). One young mother revealed to her NFP nurse that she had been tortured as a child and that she had harmed babies she took care of as an adolescent; she pleaded with her nurse to help her not do the same thing to her own baby. Supporting parents early in life leverages those protective drives that mothers and fathers are developing during this critical period defined by women's first pregnancies, births, and early caregiving.

As noted above, however, contextual factors can either support or undermine parents' care of themselves and their children. The stresses of poverty, including having insufficient income to cover survival needs (food, housing, utilities, etc.), and coping with factors like neighborhood crime, can distract parents from protecting themselves and their children. In addition, informal social systems can either amplify or buffer those adversities. Having family-members or friends who are engaged in disruptive, antisocial behavior can contribute to vulnerable parents' engaging in dysfunctional behavior themselves, while having family members and friends who are protective of the mother and child can reduce those forces that distract parents from their caregiving roles. Nurses help parents address their basic needs by linking them with other health and human services, and in engaging other family members and friends in the program, insofar as possible, to build an informal social support system that promotes maternal and child health.

Attachment theory and human ecology theory provide broad frameworks for organizing elements of an early intervention, but neither provides guidance about how to support adaptive behavioral change. For this, we turned to Bandura's self-efficacy theory (Bandura, 1977). This well-tested approach to behavioral change provides guidance to nurses about how to promote behaviors that support maternal health, fetal growth, early child health and development, and maternal economic self-sufficiency, focusing on what mothers and fathers are already doing well. The basic idea is that individuals will change their behavior to the extent that they believe change is important and they have confidence in their ability to make needed changes. Nurses guide mothers and fathers to reflect on what is important to them and to identify small, achievable objectives that will help them to accomplish their goals.

Creating Content

While the goals and core ingredients of the program have remained the same over the four-decade period during which it has been developed and tested, the specific content and methods of accomplishing NFP behavioral objectives have evolved. The program always will be a work in progress.

Elmira Trial

In the original trial of the program, conducted in Elmira, NY, and begun in 1977, David (who had become an adjunct faculty member at Cornell when funding was secured) and team (including Bob Tatelbaum and Bob Chamberlin) decided that the evidence on particular sociodemographic risks that characterize maternal vulnerabilities for poor outcomes were not definitive. So, we actively recruited women before the 24th week of gestation and who had any of these three risks: being poor (indicated primarily by their seeking free prenatal care through the local health department); unmarried; or young (<19 years of age as teen pregnancy created a risk for school dropout). In order to create a program that was not stigmatized as being for the poor or for people with problems, we made the program available to anyone in the community as long as they had no previous live births. Eighty-nine percent of those enrolled were white, 47% were less than 19 years old, 62% were unmarried, and 61% came from households headed by semi-skilled or unskilled laborers. The benefits of the program were greater for those with overlapping risks, which led us to focus recruitment in subsequent trials on those with concentrated vulnerabilities (Olds, 2002).

In planning the trial, we created a community advisory group, made up of representatives of the local medical community, public health department, department of social services, and county mental health service. Representatives of the medical community, at stages of program planning, made it clear that they would work with nurse home visitors, but not para-professional or community health workers, in serving pregnant women and young children. And while human ecology theory led us to consider including neighborhood parent-support groups to augment the nurses' work, we decided not to include this element in the intervention as women assigned to the control group would be eligible for this service, undermining the estimate of nurse-home-visiting effects. Control-group participants did receive other services through the study, however, including regular screening and referral of the child for suspected developmental problems and free transportation for regular prenatal and well-child care.

In the Elmira trial, the team had six months at the beginning of the study to identify the specific content that nurses would use in pregnancy and the first two years of the child's life, and to begin testing and adjusting features of the program based upon their work with a set of pilot families. The Elmira team brought obstetrics, pediatrics, nursing, and developmental psychology perspectives to the task, and outlined those topics that should be addressed at various stages of pregnancy and the first two years of the child's life. Program content was shaped by this outline, which was informed by an understanding of typical biological, psychological, and social changes women experience during pregnancy, the postpartum period, and phases of infant and toddler development. Nurses were encouraged to adapt this content to individual families' needs and interests. Bob Tatelbaum made the case for promoting maternal health and self-sufficiency as a separate program goal in and of itself rather than simply a means of improving child health and development.

The Elmira nurses reviewed (prior to the internet!) the most up-to-date health-education literature on modifiable factors that contributed to poor pregnancy outcomes, child health and development, and compromised maternal health and economic self-sufficiency. In organizing this literature, nurses gave particular attention to: (1) the phases of mothers' adjustment to pregnancy and anticipation of birth; and (2) parents' adjustment to the newborn and phases of caring for the child during the first two years of life.

Nurses continuously focused on maternal physical and mental health, gradually building parents' capacity to financially support themselves and their children. In all of this, program content and timing of its delivery were organized around parents' natural interests in these topics at typically-occurring phases of gestation and the first two years of life, and the role that specific influences play in shaping maternal and child health and development.

We designed the program to elicit and align with mothers' growing motivation to protect their developing child and to attune program content to that motivation. We addressed women's natural concerns about changes in their bodies during pregnancy, the prospect of giving birth, and how those concerns could be addressed with nurses' support. We aligned program content with parents' natural concerns and aspirations that unfold during this critical phase in human development, especially for those going through this experience for the first time, including caring for a vulnerable newborn and young child during periods of rapid motor, behavioral, language, and cognitive development. We selected program content on developmental epidemiologic grounds (modifiable behavioral and contextual factors that predict later health and development) and adjusted that content to parents' developing motivation to protect their child and themselves. We created a data collection system that aligned with the content and methods of program delivery to remind nurses about what content should be addressed at various developmental stages and to monitor variation in program delivery.

In the Elmira trial, nurses had caseloads that ranged between 20 and 25 families, and were scheduled to visit women every other week following registration (which occurred prior to the 24th week of gestation) and then once a week for the first six weeks after delivery, every other week through the child's fourth month of life, every three weeks through the 14th month of life, and then every four weeks until the child turned two. Nurses completed an average of nine visits during pregnancy and 23 visits from birth through child age two. Nurses visited more frequently when crises occurred. Visits lasted about 75 minutes. It became clear that nurses could not visit all families with the same frequency originally conceived, so we attempted to visit those at greatest risk in accordance with the planned schedule.

Families with fewer needs, we reasoned, could manage just fine with fewer visits.

Finally, and maybe most importantly, nurses were selected on the basis of their personal attributes—their ability to be caring, non-judgmental, and respectful. We could have exquisitely developed program content, but without employing home-visiting nurses who were empathic and non-judgmental the program would have failed. As a part of their employment interviews, we asked nurses to reflect on a series of case scenarios designed to reveal their approach to dealing with situations that might lead some to be judgmental. Nurse selection gave priority to their capacity for empathy and respect. The capacity for developing authentic, trusting, caring relationships was fundamental. Georgie was fond of reminding us that the young mothers we served "could spot a phony a mile away." Nurses from around the world have repeated nearly the same observation over and over since Georgie's original insight.

Given that this work can be highly challenging and emotionally draining, nurses are susceptible to experiencing secondary trauma. In the Elmira trial, we addressed this issue in two fundamental ways. First, nurses were paired in teams of two. They visited one another's families at periodic intervals so they would have a foundation for reflecting on the needs of their partner's highest-risk families, and they might visit their partner's families during illnesses or vacations. Second, we held weekly case conferences to discuss challenging cases as a group. We organized weekly case conferences in addition to weekly one-to-one supervision, both of which today would be thought of as reflective supervision and teamwork.

Prenatal Content

Our first overarching goal was to improve pregnancy outcomes, especially prematurity, low birthweight, and compromised neurodevelopmental functioning. We sought to do this by educating parents about the needs of the developing fetus and what mothers could do to support healthy fetal development, such as avoiding exposures to substances, prompt treatment of emerging obstetric complications, eating a nutritious diet. This work was designed to support parents' motivation for protecting their developing fetus. We elicited parents' reflections on their current behavior and what they might do to improve the life-prospects of their child.

Nurses are uniquely positioned to do this work because they can use their physical assessment skills, such as taking blood pressures in the home and checking for protein in urine or signs of edema to identify women with emerging hypertensive disorders of pregnancy to support office-based providers' care in addressing these emerging problems. Nurses taught mothers the basics of safe sex and linked them with Planned Parenthood and their primary-care providers to obtain contraceptives. Nurses also taught the basics of pregnancy physiology and fetal development to mothers and fathers, which we thought would serve as an additional incentive for behavioral change, and encouraged women to discuss their health concerns with their primary care providers during their next scheduled visit. If there were imminent concerns, such as elevated blood pressure, symptoms of genito-urinary tract infections, or signs of preterm labor, nurses urged women to call their prenatal-care providers' offices to determine whether a more immediate visit were warranted.

Finally, nurses helped women anticipate and plan for labor, delivery, and care of the newborn. During pregnancy, nurses introduced the ideas of breast feeding, effective bottle and formula feeding, bonding with the newborn, common patterns of infant behavior, including patterns of crying, early care of the child, and planning the timing of subsequent pregnancies. Nurses helped women anticipate their newborns' needs, including baby supplies, infant car seats, and safe sleeping arrangements with the child protected from undue noise or commotion.

Nurses also guided mothers and fathers to think through plans for continuing their educations, finding or continuing work following the birth of their baby, and, critically, planning the timing of their next pregnancy. Growth in education and work are enhanced to the extent that women are able to space subsequent pregnancies. Moreover, parents' care of their first child is strengthened by not having to care for two very young children at the same time. And, it turns out, that having conversations about subsequent pregnancy planning are enhanced, from women's perspectives, by nurses' raising these issues in the last few weeks before delivery. One stable, married couple informed their nurse that they wanted to have all of their children within a relatively short period of time so they could get on with their lives after child rearing. This was a wonderful reminder to us that this program is really driven by parents' visions for what they want for their lives and their children. These conversations about maternal life- course continued after delivery as mothers and fathers embraced the challenges of caring for a newborn or an inconsolable six-week old.

Where possible, we involved fathers or other family members in visits to encourage them to support maternal behavioral change and health. And, given challenges with basic survival (e.g., food insecurity, homelessness, drug abuse, family violence), nurses helped mothers make use of existing services in the community to address those needs. In all of this, nurses adapted the timing of program content to reflect the expressed interests and needs of mothers and fathers. These individualized adaptations were designed to increase program engagement, to support parents' adjustment to their new roles, and to develop a personalized vision for each family about what life might be like for themselves and their children.

Infant and Toddler Content

After delivery, nurses focused on helping parents learn the meaning of their infants' behaviors and communicative signals and learn to become sensitive, growth-promoting caregivers. Nurses reviewed existing literature on early health, development, and behavior with an eye toward helping parents recognize and respond sensitively to their newborn's signals. This work integrated human attachment theory (Bowlby, 1969) with current research and practice recommendations that aligned with our effort to promote parent-infant communication. This included helping parents with breastfeeding and the promotion of safe and well-regulated sleep patterns. In the Elmira program (before rapid discharge following delivery was standard practice), nurses visited mothers in the hospital after delivery to be with them during the discharge exam and to hear instructions from the primary care provider. Three days following discharge, the nurses conducted the Brazelton Neonatal Observation assessment (Brazelton, 1973) with parents and encouraged them to conduct the exam themselves to help parents understand their newborn's individuality and capabilities. Going forward, they encouraged sensitive, growth-promoting care through a range of activities designed to support behavioral regulation (starting with anticipating and comforting crying newborns, regulating infant sleep and feeding, and eventually helping inquisitive toddlers regulate their behavior through effective, measured limit-setting). The particular activities promoted in these areas shifted over the course of subsequent trials as new activities were developed to support parents' skills in addressing their infants' and toddlers' needs.

Nurses supported mothers and infants in a range of other ways that addressed infant health and development. Nurses continued to apply their physical assessment skills in monitoring children's physical health and growth, noting signs of compromised development and common health problems (such as fever, respiratory and skin infections, gastroenteritis, and minor trauma) and encouraged appropriate use of primary care and the emergency department when problems emerged. They helped parents create safe home environments to prevent injuries, ingestions, and exposures to environmental toxins. And, of course, nurses employed a variety of methods to promote parent support of their children's language and cognitive development, all adapted to the child's stage of development. Nurses created or relied upon publicly available materials distributed during visits to support the goals and objectives of the program and created a lending library of books for those mothers who were interested in learning more about particular topics. Nurses administered the Denver Developmental Screening (Frankenburg et al., 1971) to infants and toddlers at periodic intervals throughout the first two years of life and referred children for further evaluation and treatment when they identified potential problems. In later replications, we switched to the Ages and Stages Questionnaire (Squires, Bricker, & Potter, 1997) as a means of screening for developmental delays and guiding parents' understanding of their children's development.

Given our concern about preventing child abuse and neglect, making sure that children at imminent risk were removed from harm's way, and ensuring the nurses were complying with child maltreatment reporting laws, we set up systematic communications with the local child welfare agency. We did this to make sure that high-risk cases were reviewed anonymously with department staff and to make sure that cases were reported when warranted. Nurses were guided to let families know when they were making reports, to explain why, and to offer support to the family as they went through the child protection review process.

Memphis Trial

While many people urged us to replicate the Elmira program outside of research settings once early findings from the Elmira trial were promising, we decided not to offer the program for public investment until we had evidence that the program effects would endure and would work with minority families living in a major urban area. In 1984, David joined the Department of Pediatrics at the University of Rochester, where he formed a lasting collaboration with

Harriet Kitzman, a UR Professor of Nursing and Pediatrics. Harriet had been instrumental in launching the national nurse-practitioner movement, putting her in a unique position to integrate the NFP program more formally into the nursing profession.

After reviewing every major metropolitan area in the country as a possible site for replication of the trial, we settled on Memphis, TN. We selected Memphis because of the ease of identifying prospective participants through a free antepartum clinic for the poor sponsored by the University of Tennessee and the Memphis-Shelby County Health Department, and because healthcare for the indigent throughout the county was provided through a single system operated jointly by those entities. Moreover, all emergency care and hospitalizations of children were provided by le Bonheur Children's Hospital, which would make records of maternal and child heath relatively easy to gather and interpret, given the wide access to healthcare delivered under common protocols.

It took us four years and nine funding sources to raise funds for the Memphis trial. Those sources of funds came together in 1987 to launch the second trial of the program, which we named the Memphis New Mothers Program. For the Memphis trial, three additional co-investigators from the University of Tennessee joined the team: Dr. Kay Engelhart, Professor of Nursing, Dr. David Shafer, Professor of Obstetrics and Gynecology, and Dr. David James, Professor of Pediatrics. They were instrumental in integrating the program into the Memphis healthcare system. The program was administered through the Memphis-Shelby County Health Department and overseen by Jann Belton, a public health nurse leader in Memphis.

Given that the effects of the Elmira program on maternal and child health were more pronounced among mothers and children where there were overlapping sociodemographic risks, we concentrated recruitment in the Memphis trial on women with at least two of the following risk characteristics: unmarried, less than 12 years of education, and not working. This led to a highly disadvantaged sample, where 85% of the mothers were living in households below the federal poverty level, 98% were unmarried, and 64% were less than 19 years old. Note that families in the Memphis trial, including the control group, received developmental screening and referral services as well as free transportation for regular prenatal care. This contributed to high rates of participant enrollment: 89% of those offered participation enrolled in the trial, and retention of those randomized participants has remained high in Memphis through an 18-year follow-up. Note that we allowed women in Memphis to register through the 28th week of gestation. We changed the standard visit schedule in Memphis, and all subsequent implementations, as follows: four weekly visits following registration (to establish a relationship quickly and address pregnancy risks as early as possible); bi-weekly visits until birth; weekly visits for six weeks after birth (given the high level of change and new responsibilities mothers take on during this period); bi-weekly visits until the child reached the age of 18 months; and then, weaning mothers off the nurse's support, once-a-month visits until the child reached the age of two.

In moving the program from serving a largely white, semi-rural sample to an inner-city African- American sample, we were deeply concerned about aligning the program content and methods with the cultural beliefs and sensibilities of the families we were about to serve. To address this set of issues, we created a community advisory committee of African Americans in Memphis who provided advice about needed program adaptations. We invoked numerous surface-level adaptations, such as altering dietary recommendations to align with customary diets in the community while striving to achieve optimal nutrition for both mothers and children; making sure that images in the program materials reflected the families we were serving; and using customary language for various topics covered in the program. At a deeper level, we were concerned that in multigenerational households, where care of children may be provided in a more significant way by grandmothers or other family members, the focus on mothers may be misplaced. The grandmothers in our advisory group told us, however, to keep the focus on the mothers as they needed to learn the skills provided by the nurses. As in the Elmira program, we made significant efforts, nevertheless, to engage fathers, grandmothers, and other caregivers in an effort to create shared approaches to caregiving among those responsible for the child.

Harriet was instrumental in transforming the Elmira program into a format that aligned with nursing education and practice that continues to shape program design today. One of Harriet's many insights was that in order to build a foundation for nurses' learning the program and for our disseminating it reliably, it would need to align with the way nurses are taught to practice, with a particular focus on the "Nursing Process" (Orlando, 1961, 1972), that is, assessing parents' needs, exploring with parents the extent to which the nurse's assessments are correct from parents' perspectives, setting in motion a plan of action in concert with parents, and evaluating those actions. The essence of the program remained the same as that tested in Elmira, but it was strengthened by building upon generations of nursing science and practice that has led nursing to be the most trusted profession in the US for generations (Brenan, 2018).

Harriet's insight was to take the Elmira program and break it into the following domains: (1) maternal health, (2) maternal role, (3) maternal life-course, (4) family and friends, and (5) environmental health in a way that built upon the underlying epidemiology and theory of the Elmira program. These program domains have continued to organize the nurses' work to this day, with the recent addition of an explicit domain that, consistent with the Elmira program design, encompasses nurses' orchestrating families' use of needed health and human services. In addition, nursing scientists had developed theories of human caring that had become fundamental to all of nursing practice (Watson, 1979). As a result of Harriet's work, caring became an explicit feature of the program, which had been fundamental to the Elmira program, but not explicitly identified.

Another of Harriet's insights was that the program would be replicated more reliably if it were divided into a visit-by-visit structure, with particular content recommended in the five program domains at specific visits throughout pregnancy, infancy, and toddlerhood. This approach differed from the one employed in Elmira, where nurses were guided by an outline of content organized around phases of prenatal and infant/toddler development, and encouraged to adapt it to individual families' concerns and interests. The visit-by-visit structure set in motion in Memphis was designed to help ensure consistency for mothers and nurses, but with clear guidance that nurses adapt program content and dosage to the needs of families on a visit-to-visit, moment-to-moment basis.

Moreover, to elicit mother/caregiver engagement in targeted behavioral change, Harriet transformed the program content into "facilitators," that is, a set of interesting questions and game-like formats designed to elicit participant reflection on every topic covered under the five program domains most relevant during specific stages of pregnancy, postpartum, infancy, and toddlerhood. Those reflections were used as the starting point for behavioral change, organized around program goals and objectives. In all of this, nurses educated mothers, fathers, and other caregivers to promote maternal and child health and development, grounded in their desire to see their child thrive. Nurses helped them develop small achievable objectives and celebrated successes at every visit. We gave mothers notebooks with new informational materials added to the notebook at each visit, which mothers kept for reference.

Mothers were observed sitting on their front steps using these materials to educate other family members, friends, and neighbors who might benefit from them.

Finally, we invited Kathy Barnard, a professor of maternal-child nursing from the University of Washington, to join the Memphis team. Our team was constantly reviewing the literature on maternal and child health to identify new methods of promoting maternal and child health and was delighted to see that Kathy had developed a measure of parent-child interaction—the NCAST (Nursing Child Assessment Satellite Training)—which we introduced as a clinical component of the program. The NCAST Feeding and Teaching Scales were a natural extension of the program's focus on supporting sensitive, growth- promoting parental caregiving. The integration of NCAST into NFP was one of the first systematic methods of promoting early parenting that relied upon observations of parent-child interaction as the starting point for education. All nurses were trained in the NCAST and were encouraged to integrate it into their practice when discussing child development.

Denver Trial

In 1993, David was recruited to the University of Colorado to conduct the third trial of the program and to develop the Prevention Research Center for Family and Child Health in the Department of Pediatrics in the CU School of Medicine. Ruth

O'Brien, professor of nursing at the CU College of Nursing, joined the investigative team to bring an additional nursing science perspective to this work. The Denver trial was designed to test the relative impact of the program when delivered by nurses versus community health workers; both of these groups were compared to a control group offered child developmental screening and referral services. The Denver sample included a large portion of Hispanics. The inclusion of Hispanics in the Denver trial broadened the program's solid foundation, further generalizing its positive effects to large portions of the population in need in US society.

The nursing supervisor in the Denver trial was Pilar Baca, MSN. Pilar led work on adapting the program to Latinx culture, including translating all program guidelines and materials into Spanish. All program materials were reviewed and adapted to ensure that they reflected images familiar to Latinx families and that nutritional, health behavior, and childrearing recommendations were brought into alignment with the prevailing sensibilities of Latinx families. Some Latinx families, for example, especially recent immigrants, place considerable value on child behavioral compliance with rules, which shaped the way limit-setting was framed with Latinx families. Pilar also brought to this effort a skill in distilling key features of the program into aphorisms that are easily remembered and that helped deepen the culture of the program. They include "The mother is the expert in her own life;" "Follow the mother's heart's desire;" "Only a small change is needed;" "Focus on strengths;" and "Focus on solutions." In addition to developing more program "facilitators" to help address issues that new mothers and fathers often encounter, Pilar led the development of additional visit-by-visit program guidelines. She and Ruth O'Brien augmented the self-efficacy foundations of the program by adding Solution-Focused approaches to working with families (O'Brien and Baca, 1997). This approach was later integrated with the emerging field of Motivational Interviewing (Miller & Rollnick, 1991). These approaches represent clinically sophisticated methods of eliciting mother's primary motivations—"heart's desire," by "focusing on strengths," and to support behavioral change. This approach provides a systematic way of eliciting parents' deepest motivations, which nurses rely on to support and guide parents' efforts to protect their children and promote self-efficacy in accomplishing their other goals.

Refining, Expanding, Disseminating

After nearly 20 years focused on developing the program and its evidentiary foundations, we began to consider invitations to replicate the program outside of research settings.

US Community Replication

In 1996, we accepted an invitation to replicate the program in high-crime communities under an initiative sponsored by the US Justice Department.

The early community replication work was managed through a new center (the National Center for Children, Families, and Communities) we created in the University of Colorado School of Nursing with a significant investment from the Robert Wood Johnson Foundation. Pilar continued to serve as director of nursing in the newly created NCCFC. In this capacity, she further articulated reflective supervision in the model as a natural extension of the program's focus on deep clinical supervision that aligns with its core components (Gibbs, 1981). In laying the groundwork for community replication, we developed a model that spelled out nurse-education, organizational, and community conditions needed to promote reliable reproduction of program effects in new community settings (Olds, 2002; Olds et al., 2003). David Racine and Gerry Sommerville from Replication and Program Strategies, a non-profit based in Philadelphia, provided great insights that helped us to develop our model of community replication. The work we had conducted in the original trials provided a foundation for having a reasonably well articulated program when we began community replication. During the conduct of the trials, we had built an information system that was integrated into the program so that key features of program implementation and maternal and child outcomes could be monitored in the process of community replication.

In 2003, once it became clear that there was considerable interest in new communities' investing in the program (with the program operating in nearly 250 US counties), we created a separate non-profit devoted to further expanding it throughout the US. The program was then given its current name: Nurse-Family Partnership. This name, we think, reflects its underlying sprit of collaboration between the family and nurse. It is important to note that the University of Colorado owns the NFP intellectual property and gives the NFP non-profit a royalty-free license to replicate the program—in accordance with 19 core model elements constructed to help ensure that the program is replicated with essential fidelity to the model tested in the original trials. These elements cover a range of program features, including target population characteristics, program staffing and training, adherence to program content and methods of delivery, caseload size, supervision, data collection requirements, organization capacity, and evidence of community commitment.

Elly Yost was an early director of the NFP national nursing department who later joined the CU Department of Pediatrics as an instructor at the PRC, where she oversees work focused on formatively developing innovations to improve the underlying NFP model and its implementation in community settings. Elly has convened an innovations advisory committee composed of over 120 NFP nurses, supervisors, and agency administrators devoted to strengthening the program model and its implementation. These volunteers are passionately committed to making the program as strong and efficient as it can be.

We also have developed a model for improving the NFP in community practice (Olds et al., 2013). One of the innovations set in motion during community replication consists of a new method for nurses to use in observing and supporting early parental care of the child. This new method is known as DANCE (Dyadic Assessment of Nurse Caregiver Experiences) and is led by Dr. Nancy Donelan-McCall at the PRC. DANCE was developed in response to difficulties nurses reported in learning and using the NCAST procedure to promote parent-child interaction. DANCE consists of scales that apply to very young children and that are linked directly to program "facilitators" designed to promote parent-child interaction. The scales are grounded in reviews of the literature on influences on child development, infant mental health, and parent-child interaction. Studies of video-taped interactions of participants in the Denver trial found that DANCE assessments over the first two years of life are predictive of children's directly-measured cognitive, language, and academic abilities during preschool and early elementary school years.

In addition, given that program effects in the Elmira trial on reducing state-verified reports of child abuse and neglect were attenuated in households characterized by moderate to severe intimate partner violence (Eckenrode et al., 2000), Drs. Susan Jack and Harriet MacMillan at McMaster University in Canada led a carefully conducted formative effort to develop nurse education and clinical skills to more effectively address IPV in the context of home visits. This augmentation of the model was tested in a cluster-based RCT that compared NFP sites delivering the program as usual to NFP sites that were taught to deliver the IPV intervention. While it had no effects on maternal reports of IPV and quality of life (Jack et al., 2019), nurses who received IPV education reported greater knowledge of IPV and confidence in addressing it. We are in the midst of conducting additional analyses to help sort out these findings.

We also tested an intervention designed to increase participant retention by encouraging nurses to adapt program content and dosage more completely to meet mothers' needs. We found that participant retention was reduced in community replication compared to the original trials, and that lower retention was linked to some nurses delivering the program with strict adherence to the visit-by-visit guidelines as opposed to adapting content and methods to families' needs. Nurses who adapted the program had higher rates of retention (O'Brien et al., 2012). This retention intervention produced promising findings in a cluster-based RCT (Olds et al., 2015) and has reinforced our commitment to guiding nurses in eliciting mothers' "heart's desire" and adapting program content and dosage to align with those desires.

NFP nurses have been guided since the Elmira trial to adapt program content and dosage to the needs of families on an individual basis, but until recently there has been no systematic approach for guiding those adaptations. This is now addressed through the STAR (Strengths and Risk) Framework, a systematic way for nurses to organize their assessments of individual and family strengths, and to characterize proximal and distal risks that affect maternal and child health. Proximal risks are those that have rather direct impacts on maternal and child health (e.g., substance use, depression, intellectual functioning), while distal risks indirectly influence maternal and child functioning (e.g., having insufficient money to pay rent, transportation challenges, friends involved in the drug trade). These strengths and risks are organized in accordance with program model domains, the underlying theories that have guided program design since Elmira, and the "nursing process."

Moreover, formative work is now being conducted in 31 sites to develop a version of the program for women with previous live births who have overlapping behavioral and psychosocial risks. This formative modification of the model builds upon work begun with indigenous populations in Australia and the US, but requires a randomized clinical trial before being delivered on a full-scale basis, given that all of the original trials were conducted with women who had no previous live births. A complementary initiative is under way to strengthen nurses' skills in addressing substance misuse, with a particular focus on serving those who are in treatment. This narrow focus on those either with or at risk of developing substance use disorders warrants testing in randomized clinical trials.

Today, the NFP National nursing department is led by Kate Siegrist, who is focused on ensuring high caliber nurse education and consultation to make sure that nurses are practicing at the top of their skill set in addressing the full range of factors that challenge maternal and child health. Kate has led work to create even greater alignment between the NFP nursing program and the American Nurses Association and Public Health Nurses standards for nurses delivering the NFP. Under Kate's leadership and in concert with Elly, the NFP has recently developed an app used by mothers and nurses to track mothers' growth in establishing and accomplishing their individual goals. The "Goal Mama" app is being carefully evaluated and adjusted to ensure its functionality and use among mothers enrolled in the program.

In addition, the number of program "facilitators" has grown since Harriet introduced this approach in the late 1980s. Today, hundreds of "facilitators" are organized into an electronic, searchable database that nurses use to find guidance in addressing the unique needs of individual mothers and families throughout the two-and-a-half-year program. Nurses have confidence that if families need something, it is highly likely to be found in the NFP "facilitator" database.

International Replication

While the US national office managed replication of the NFP in the US, the PRC at the University of Colorado began considering invitations to replicate the program outside of the US. International replication was undertaken with deep appreciation for the need to adapt the program to other cultures and contexts, and to make the conduct of independent RCTs a condition for replication when feasible. As with US replication, there are a set of "Core Model Elements" that needed to be preserved for the University to grant use of its intellectual property. One of the earliest international replications took place in the Netherlands, starting with the conduct of a randomized trial with highly vulnerable families, which found effects comparable to key findings in the US trials. The Dutch effort did not include the development of an information system that could be used to monitor program implementation and guide improvements, however. Given that we could not be certain of quality program replication, we did not continue NFP in the Netherlands. Similarly, we supported the development and testing of the program in Germany, but the German effort included non-nurses as home visitors in some settings, so we did not continue licensing the program there.

We have received numerous invitations to set up the program in low- and middle-income countries, where resources are scarce and political environments unstable. We have chosen not to invest resources in those contexts so far because we have been less confident that the program would gain traction in those settings. We were deeply interested in evaluating the program in dramatically different cultural contexts, however, so when we were invited to develop the program in aboriginal communities in Australia, we accepted the invitation. We did so because it was clear that the Australian government was committed for the long-haul in supporting NFP adaptation, building community ownership, and imbuing the program with sufficient resources to give it a chance to gain traction in these diverse settings. A government advisory committee indicated at the beginning of the Australian effort that in order for the program to be culturally appropriate in remote indigenous communities, nurses would need to serve all women, not only those with no previous live births. They also advised that nurses would need to be paired with community health workers who would introduce the program to families and others in an effort to create cultural safety. We gladly agreed to these modifications in the program model. Today, the NFP operates in 13 aboriginal led community health settings throughout the country. While the program is not going to be tested in the form of an RCT, given that depriving some families of the service would be considered culturally inappropriate, a well-conducted quasi-experimental evaluation has found effects that align with the US trials (Segal et al., 2018). Additional evaluative work is being planned.

A similar approach to serving indigenous populations is being used in serving American Indian and Alaskan Native populations in North America, including British Columbia, Canada. In all of this work, we were uncertain whether the program would resonate to dramatically different populations with dramatically different histories and cultures. The essence of the model that aligns it with these populations is best expressed by an American Indian spiritual leader who told David that the program aligns with his peoples' aspirations because "Children are gifts of the Great Creator." In Alice Springs, Australia, the program was blessed with a smoke ceremony as part of its inauguration in that community. As human beings, we are wired to protect and promote the wellbeing of our offspring. This is a fundamental insight that, if we listen carefully, can be relied upon to help ensure that the program will gain traction if communities and individual families are engaged in a respectful way that reflects our shared humanity.

The first phase of a randomized trial of the program in England produced disappointing findings, perhaps because existing health visitors and midwives serving adolescents were told which families were in the control group, apparently leading them to provide more intensive services to the control group than they would under "usual care." Nevertheless, the program currently is operating in 80 communities in England and every community in Scotland, as well as high-need communities in Northern Ireland. A follow-up study of the English trial is in the pipeline.

Preliminary work is being conducted in Norway and in Bulgaria (where it is primarily serving Roma families) to formatively develop an adapted version of the program and to lay the groundwork for a rigorous evaluation. In addition, a province-wide initiative is being undertaken in British Columbia where the provincial government has invested in a large-scale RCT, with appropriate adaptations made to local health and human service contexts, including to First Nations (indigenous) communities served in the province. The results of the BC trial for the prenatal phase will be published soon.

The success of the international work has depended significantly on our engaging skilled nursing leaders from the UK and Canada in supporting broader international replication. After establishing the program in their own countries, several nursing leaders went on to support NFP international replication through the University of Colorado. Kate Billingham, Deputy Chief Nursing Officer in the UK Department of Health, served as the first director of the Family-Nurse-Partnership (as it is called there) in England. Kate transitioned to serve as the first director of international replication of the Nurse-Family Partnership. Ann Rowe, who served as the first director of clinical operations for the Family-Nurse- Partnership in England has gone on to serve as the lead consultant guiding NFP international replication in new contexts. Debbie Sheehan, a nurse leader in Ontario, Canada, was instrumental in establishing the program in Hamilton, Ontario and guiding its development in British Columbia; Debbie supported international replication of the program for several years. Gail Trotter, a nurse leader who led development of the program in Scotland, has recently moved on to serve as a consultant to the PRC supporting the program. The clinical and leadership skills of these nurses have been critical in laying the foundation for quality program replication in growing international contexts.

As of this writing, the world is coping with the COVID-19 pandemic. Nurses delivering the program around the world are resorting to the use of telephone and other electronic means of conducting visits with participating families. Fortunately, Elly Yost had led an initiative to determine the feasibility of using "telehealth" modalities in delivering the program and developed clinical guidance on the use of these methods to conduct visits. We are just at the beginning of this crisis and NFP is adjusting its information system to focus on families' needs during this crisis and to monitor families' course of coping with the virus and its societal and economic impact. Those families living on the margins are at greatest risk. They either do not have cell phone access or have unstable access; their sources of income are more vulnerable; and they live in crowded housing where the spread of infection is most likely to occur. NFP programs around the world are sharing resources and insights about how to confront this crisis.

Lessons Learned

The success of NFP can be attributed to four fundamental features that have guided its development. First, its grounding in theory has helped shape, in broad terms, what nurses are going to focus on in their work with families. The program's theories cover the map in addressing broad swaths of behavior and context that shape successful adaptation to parenting and promotion of child health and development. Second, the program's grounding in epidemiology and its continuous updating to align with the latest evidence on risks and protective factors has guided the development of new program content, which ensures that NFP will continue to operate at the cutting edge of science and clinical practice. Third, its reliance on a well-developed information system allows its leaders to monitor its performance. And fourth, NFP leaders' commitment to disciplined, research-based improvement efforts means that the model and its delivery will always be a work in progress

One of the key lessons learned from this work is that the enduring success of the program can be attributed to its alignment with our shared human drive to protect our children, and that the success of our efforts can be explained by nurses' developing caring, respectful relationships with mothers and other caregivers which elicit that drive and enable it to be used in a focused way to achieve cumulative small steps toward what matters most to mothers and other caregivers. By working with mothers during pregnancy and the early years of the child's life, we are capitalizing on unique opportunities presented at a critical period in human development—when changes in maternal roles and neuroendocrine systems shape maternal caregiving skills going forward, and when fetal and infant development are particularly sensitive to a range of toxic and growth-promoting exposures.

Critically, the program is integrated with nursing, which builds upon caring, holistic assessment and evidence-based practice as the foundation for effective health promotion. Nurses have the education to address critical aspects of maternal and child physical-health, behavioral-health, and environmental-health that, during pregnancy and the early years of life, shape the life prospects of mothers, fathers, and children for decades following the first child's birth.

In all of this, there is value in creating a program that is both structured and designed to be adapted to individual mothers, other caregivers, cultures, and contexts—while retaining its core elements. Adherence to these elements is crucial, but there are program elements that do not work as well as they need to and factors that will interfere with its implementation in some settings, elements that we will continue to seek to understand and improve. If we remember what matters most, and approach this work with humility and respect for those with whom we partner, we can make a growing difference in the lives of vulnerable mothers, children, and families.

Acknowledgements

We would like to dedicate this chapter to the memory of Harriet Kitzman. And we wish to thank the thousands of nurses and families who have inspired us, guided us, and challenged us to make this program even better going forward.

References

Ainsworth, M. D., Blehar, M. C., Waters, E., & Wall, S. (1978). *Patterns of attachment: A psychological study of the strange situation*. Hillsdale, NJ: Lawrence Erlbaum, Associates.

Bandura, A. (1977). Self-efficacy: Toward a unifying theory of behavioral change. *Psychological Review*, *84*(2), 191–215.

Bowlby, J. (1969). *Attachment and loss, 1. Attachment*. Basic Books.

Brazelton, T. B. (1973). *Neonatal behavioral assessment scale*. Clinics in Developmental Medicine No. 50. William Heinemann Medical Books Ltd., J.B. Lippincott Co.

Brenan, M. (2018, December 20). Nurses again outpace other professions for honesty, ethics. *Gallup*. Retrieved from https://news.gallup.com/poll/245597/nurses-again-outpace-professions-honesty-ethics.aspx

Bronfenbrenner, U. (1979). *The ecology of human development: Experiments by nature and design*. Cambridge, MA: Harvard University Press.

Eckenrode, J., Ganzel, B., Henderson, C. R., Jr., Smith, E., Olds, D. L., Powers, J., Cole, R., Kitzman, H., & Sidora, K. (2000). Preventing child abuse and neglect with a program of nurse home visitation: The limiting effects of domestic violence. *JAMA*, *284*(11), 1385–1391.

Frankenburg, W. K., Camp, B. W., Van Natta, P. A., & Demersseman, J. A. (1971). Reliability and stability of the Denver Developmental Screening Test. *Child Development*, *42*(5), 1315–1325.

Jack, S. M., Boyle, M., McKee, C., Ford-Gilboe, M., Wathen, C. N., Scribano, P., … MacMillan, H. L. (2019). Effect of addition of an intimate partner violence intervention to a nurse home visitation program on maternal quality of life: A randomized clinical trial. *JAMA*, *321*(16), 1576–1585.

Miller, W. R., & Rollnick, S. (1991). *Motivational interviewing: Preparing people to change addictive behavior*. New York: The Guilford Press.

O'Brien, R. A., & Baca, R. P. (1997). Application of solution-focused interventions to nurse home visitation for pregnant women and parents of young children. *The Journal of Community Psychology*, *25*(1), 47–57.

O'Brien, R. A., Moritz, P., Luckey, D. W., McClatchey, M. W., Ingoldsby, E. M., & Olds, D. L. (2012). Mixed methods analysis of participant attrition in the nurse-family partnership. *Prevention Science*, *13*(3), 219–228.

Olds, D., Donelan-McCall, N., O'Brien, R., MacMillan, H., Jack, S., Jenkins, T., ... Beeber, L. (2013). Improving the nurse-family partnership in community practice. *Pediatrics*, *132*, S110–S117.

Olds, D. L. (2002). Prenatal and infancy home visiting by nurses: From randomized trials to community replication. *Prevention Science*, *3*(3), 153–172.

Olds, D. L., Baca, P., McClatchey, M., Ingoldsby, E. M., Luckey, D. W., Knudtson, M. D., ... Ramsey, M. (2015). Cluster randomized controlled trial of intervention to increase participant retention and completed home visits in the nurse-family partnership. *Prevention Science*, *16*(6), 778–788.

Olds, D. L., Hill, P., O'Brien, R., Racine, D., & Moritz, P. (2003). Taking preventive intervention to scale: The nurse-family partnership. *Cognitive and Behavioral Practice*, *10*(4), 278–290.

Orlando, I. J. (1961). *The dynamic nurse-patient relationship: Function, process mid principles*. GP Putnam's Sons, 31–60.

Orlando, I. J. (1972). The discipline and teaching of nursing process. In J. George (Ed.), *Nursing theories: The base for professional nursing practice*. Appleton & Lange.

Segal, L., Nguyen, H., Gent, D., Hampton, C., & Boffa, J. (2018). Child protection outcomes of the Australian nurse family partnership program for aboriginal infants and their mothers in Central Australia. *PLOS ONE*, *13*(12), e0208764.

Social Programs that Work. (2020). *What works in social policy?* Retrieved from https://evidencebasedprograms.org/

Squires, J., Bricker, D., & Potter, L. (1997). Revision of a parent-completed developmental screening tool: Ages and stages questionnaires. *Journal of Pediatric Psychology*, *22*(3), 313–328.

Sumner, G. A., & Spietz, A. (1995). *NCAST caregiver/parent-child interaction teaching manual*. NCAST Publications.

Swain, J. E., Kim, P., Spicer, J., Ho, S. S., Dayton, C. J., Elmadih, A., & Abel, K. M. (2014). Approaching the biology of human parental attachment: Brain imaging, oxytocin and coordinated assessments of mothers and fathers. *Brain Research*, *1580*, 78–101.

van't Veer, A. E., Thijssen, S., Witteman, J., van IJzendoorn, M. H., & Bakermans-Kranenburg, M. J. (2019). Exploring the neural basis for paternal protection: An investigation of the neural response to infants in danger. *Social Cognitive and Affective Neuroscience*, *14*(4), 447–457.

Watson, J. (1979). *Nursing: The philosophy and science of caring*. Little, Brown.

Chapter 13

The New Beginnings Program for Divorced and Separated Families

Sharlene A. Wolchik and Irwin N. Sandler

The New Beginnings Program (NBP) is a relatively brief parenting program for divorced and separated families that has been shown to have positive short-term effects on children's mental health problems in three randomized controlled trials. Long-term follow-ups showed positive program effects not only on mental health problems, substance use, and risky sexual behavior but competencies, such as adaptive coping, grades, and attitudes toward parenting six years and 15 years after participation. In this chapter, we describe the impetus for developing the program, its underlying small theory, and the methods we used to develop the program content and activities. We then discuss those aspects of the program that worked well and those that did not and how we used the lessons learned in each trial to refine the program and maximize its public health impact.

Starting Point

Our interest in divorce began in 1982 when Sharlene was supervising second-year clinical psychology graduate students. She noticed that about half the families seeking services in the clinic were divorced or in the process of getting divorced. Having been trained to use evidence-based interventions whenever possible, she turned to the literature for guidance. She discovered that the existing research focused primarily on either characterizing differences in the adjustment of children in divorced and married families or identifying risk and protective factors for divorced families. What was most striking to Sharlene was that there was almost no research from the child's perspective. At that time, Irwin was using life-events methodology to assess the array of stressors individuals experienced, including those experienced by children in high risk situations. After learning about this approach, Sharlene talked with Irwin about identifying stressful events from the perspective of children in divorced families. That 30-minute conversation that took place nearly 40 years ago was the beginning of an incredible collaboration that is still going strong today.

In our first project, we developed a life-events measure to "unpack" children's experience of parental divorce. We then conducted several studies to assess the influence of potentially malleable risk and protective factors on mental health problems. Two other individuals played invaluable roles in this early phase. Sandy Braver, a faculty member in our department, provided statistical expertise and Susan Westover, an advanced graduate student, brought exceptional clinical insight. Their personal experiences with divorce gave them a perspective that enriched our work. Susan's passion for clinical work led her to develop a parenting-after-divorce program that served as the foundation for the New Beginnings Program (NBP).

Underlying Theory

When we developed the NBP, there were very few experimental evaluations of programs for divorced families. Only one (Pedro-Carroll & Cowen, 1985) of three evaluations of a child-focused program found significant program effects on children's mental health problems. The only existing evaluation of a parent-focused program, which aimed to facilitate children's adjustment by enhancing mothers' identity development, social support, and parenting was not found to improve children's mental health problems (Stolberg & Garrison, 1985).

Our approach to program development differed from that used by others in several ways. First, our decisions about the nature and content of the program were explicitly based on the research we and others had conducted on the potentially modifiable correlates of children's post-divorce adjustment problems. Our review showed that the correlates with the strongest empirical support, such as parent-child relationship quality and effective discipline, were within parents' rather than children's control. Thus, we chose parents as change agents, a decision supported by research showing that parents were effective change agents with other at-risk populations. Second, in addition to drawing from the overarching person-environment transactional model and the risk and protective factor theoretical framework, we formulated a "small theory" (i.e., logic model) that articulated the processes through which the program was expected to improve children's outcomes. We integrated a test of this theory in each trial we conducted to assess whether the program changed the targeted processes and whether change in those processes accounted for change in children's problems. Third, when possible, we selected strategies that had been shown in previous research to change these processes. Fourth, we built in strategies to increase the likelihood that parents would use the skills in their daily lives, both during and after the program.

To maximize the chances of impacting significant public health outcomes, multiple factors were targeted based on evidence that they were related to children's mental health problems and were modifiable. In reviewing the literature on children's post-divorce adjustment, we found sufficient support to include the following potentially modifiable factors in the NBP: residential parent-child relationship quality, effective discipline, the frequency of non-residential

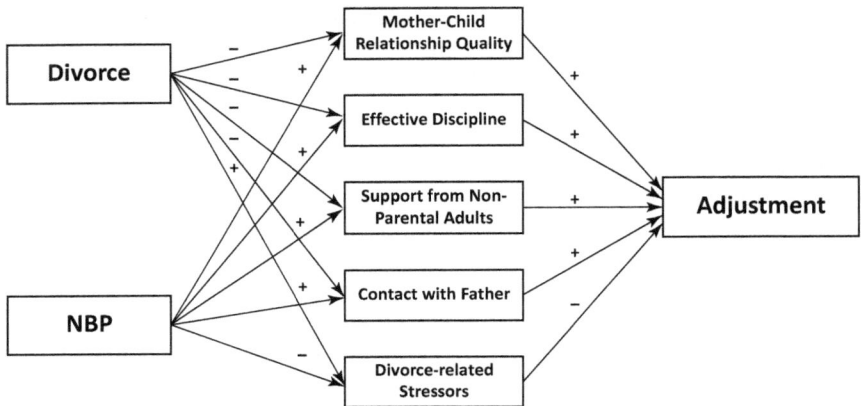

Figure 13.1 Small theory of the New Beginnings Program

parent-child contact, support from non-parental adults, and negative divorce-related stressors including interparental conflict (See Wolchik et al., 1993 for support for these factors). We think of these factors as putative mediators because we expected that changing them would affect children's mental health problems. As shown in Figure 13.1, in our small theory, we conceptualized divorce as leading to decreases in residential parent-child relationship quality, effective discipline, non-residential parent-child contact, support from non-parental adults, and an increase in divorce-related stressors. We hypothesized that the program would affect these putative mediators, which would lead to reductions in children's mental health problems.

Specifics of the NBP

The theoretical orientation of the NBP change strategies is cognitive-behavioral. When possible, we relied on change strategies described in the treatment literature on children's mental health problems and parenting programs. For the components that targeted increasing the quality of the mother-child relationship and helping children cope with divorce-related stressors, we based our strategies on those described by Guerney (1978) and Forehand and McMahon (1981) as well as our clinical experiences and intuition. For example, we adapted Forehand and McMahon's Child's Game to be appropriate for children between the ages of 8 and 15. Guerney's (1978) communication strategies formed the base for the good listening skills we taught. Based on our clinical intuition, we developed Family Fun Time, an activity designed to help promote a new family identity and enhance positive relationships in the family. To bolster effective discipline, we employed strategies used by Patterson

(1975) and Forehand and McMahon (1981). Mothers learned to "catch 'em [their children] being good" for positive behavior, use age-appropriate expectations, communicate their expectations clearly, and develop behavior change plans to reduce misbehaviors. We built on Novaco's (1975) research on anger management to help mother cope with their emotions and quickly end conflictual interactions with their former spouses that occurred in front of their children. We instructed mothers to anticipate that a conflict might occur, use self-talk to remind themselves of the importance of not fighting in front of the children and calm down and then to say, several times if necessary, that they would not talk about this issue in front of the children and suggest a time when the issue could be discussed in private. We drew on Marlatt and Gordon's (1985) work on relapse prevention in the area of substance use to help parents recognize that setbacks are not atypical and identify strategies to help them persist in using the program skills, such as using reminders. Finally, we relied on our clinical experience and intuition to craft practical strategies to increase father-child contact and support from non-parental adults. For father contact, mothers identified obstacles to visitation and leaders helped them develop strategies to remove the obstacles. To increase support from non-parental adults, mothers completed a social network assessment, made plans to increase contact between supportive adults and their children, and problem solved potential barriers. The number of sessions we allotted to each putative mediator depended on how strongly it was supported by the correlational research and how many sessions we thought were needed to teach the skill.

We decided to use a group rather than an individual format to keep costs as low as possible and promote parents learning from each other and supporting each other's use of the program skills. Our decision to include only mothers in the efficacy trials, rather than mothers and fathers, was based on what we learned during a clinical pilot of a combined group. Not only did we have a few parents who were outwardly hostile toward the opposite-sex group members, there were also some unwelcome requests from some participants to others for contact outside of group. This was an experience we did not want to repeat! So, in the efficacy trials, we focused only on mothers because, at that time, the vast majority of children lived with their mothers after divorce and groups for fathers were not practically viable. As father's post-divorce involvement in children's lives increased over the years, we developed and evaluated a father version, which had positive effects on children's mental health problems.

The program in the first trial consisted of 10 group sessions (1.75 hours each) and two one-hour individual sessions between the group leader and parent. The majority of the sessions focused on parenting (five on mother-child relationship quality, two on discipline). The individual sessions focused on helping mothers use the skills at home with their children more effectively. Maintenance was promoted throughout the program. Parents were expected to use the skills taught in earlier sessions along with the new skill taught that week and encouraged to set regular times for the activities of Family Fun Time and One-on-One Time so that they became part of the family's routines. The last two sessions addressed other ways to keep using the program skills, such as putting reminders about the program skills in prominent places, reviewing the workbooks, and checking in with friends or relatives about using the program skills.

We decided to start with activities to increase mother-child relationship quality rather than discipline, which was of more pressing interest to some mothers for three reasons. First, the activities such as Family Fun Time and One-on-One Time were relatively easy to learn and use, so the mothers usually implemented them with their children. These activities in themselves often led to positive changes in relationship quality and children's behaviors. Second, because these activities usually led to improvements, we thought they would provide motivation to try other program activities. Third, we expected that improving relationship quality might reduce some misbehaviors so there would be less need to address them later in the program.

In designing our sessions, we used Benjamin Franklin's perspective on learning as a guide, "Tell me and I may forget. Show me and I may remember. Involve me and I will learn." We used active learning principles to maximize involvement and promote learning and strove to make the sessions as engaging as possible. We presented the didactic material in a conversational, interactive style, allowed time for parents to share their experiences, lectured as little as possible, and often asked questions or led exercises to make key teaching points. Through these activities, many of our intended messages emerged through mothers' own ideas, and then were discussed and highlighted as a group. By working in this way, the mothers were more likely to "own" the material because it emerged from their own thinking and discussion rather than from a group leader telling them what to do. For example, in the component on discipline, we started by asking mothers to reflect on what makes discipline so difficult after divorce, had them complete a self-assessment of their discipline style, and asked them to brainstorm what children likely learn from different styles.

Based on successful parenting programs with other populations, we knew that a key to reducing children's problems was getting parents to use the skills on a regular basis and so we employed several strategies to promote skill use. First, we provided what we thought was a compelling rationale for the importance of using each skill after divorce. For example, in introducing effective discipline, we provided the following reasons why effective discipline would be helpful: It reassures children that their world is more predictable. It leads to more cooperation. It reduces stress for mothers and children and decreases negative cycles between them. In the effectiveness trial, we also used video testimonials in which parents talked about how the skill benefitted their family. Second, leaders role played the skills in the first trial and we used leader role plays and video demonstrations in the latter two trials. For some skills, such as good listening, we showed videos of actors demonstrating the skill poorly first and then correctly next, which we hoped would help mothers identify the key elements of effective skill use. Third, in each session, the mothers practiced the new skill and received feedback about what they did well and what they could do differently. Fourth, the importance of using the skills was emphasized throughout the program. Parents frequently heard the program motto: "Homework is the program." Also, leaders consistently attributed reported changes in children's behaviors to changes in parents' behaviors to build mothers' self-efficacy and increase motivation to use the skills. Fifth, 20 to 25 minutes of each session were devoted to reviewing the use of skills over the past week and troubleshooting problems. Leaders reinforced mothers for trying the skills and making small gains and used a collaborative approach to develop solutions for difficulties. To increase accountability, mothers recorded whether they used each skill and how it went. Leaders reviewed these forms and provided many comments that reinforced the mothers' efforts and suggested ways to employ the skills more often or more effectively. When leaders returned the forms from the previous week at the beginning of each session, mothers eagerly read each and every comment. Finally, to ensure that mothers had an opportunity to learn all the skills, we provided short make-up sessions right before each session for those who had been absent the prior session. Throughout the program, leaders promoted group cohesion by pointing out similarities in mothers' experiences and reinforcing mothers for helping other mothers problem solve. We felt that group cohesion would increase the effects of the support mothers provided to each other for skill use. Leaders also provided hope by telling mothers that it often took time for changes in children's behavior to occur and sharing stories of the changes other mothers had seen through the program. Providing hope and promoting cohesion were seen as essential because the program requires a great deal of work, and it often takes some time before mothers see the results of their efforts.

Given that the central goal of this trial was to evaluate whether the program, when delivered as designed, affected children's mental health outcomes, fidelity was a high priority. We used multiple approaches to maximize fidelity. The content and format of all sessions were described in very detailed outlines, which leaders were expected to use as they delivered the sessions. Each outline included a section that described common difficulties in using the skills and solutions for them. After the first trial, we wondered if less detailed outlines might be easier for leaders to follow and did a small clinical pilot with abbreviated session outlines. Although the groups seemed to work well, the feedback from the leaders was consistent and clear: They wanted more rather than less detail in the outlines. So, moving forward, we used very detailed outlines. Also, leaders received intensive training (30 hours) that included readings and didactic information about children's post-divorce adjustment and the theoretical and empirical bases for the program, videotapes from a pilot of the program, and role play of session material. Further, to make preparation and delivery more manageable, two leaders conducted each group. Finally, we provided weekly training (one hour) and weekly supervision (1.5 hours). During training, leaders role-played activities in the upcoming session so that they felt prepared and confident. Parallel to the process we wanted leaders to use with parents, supervision aimed to build a sense of self-efficacy by reinforcing specific positive behaviors and helping leaders develop solutions to the difficulties they experienced.

We recruited families using a random sampling of publicly available court records of divorces with children, media articles, and school presentations. Mothers were sent a letter and received a call about participating. This method of recruitment was very time consuming and effortful.

Refining the NBP

We learned a lot from the first trial! By collecting extensive process and outcome data, we were able to assess whether the components were implemented as intended, whether change occurred in the putative mediators and outcome variables, and whether changes in the mediators accounted for change in children's behavior problems. These data allowed us to test the small theory of the program.

On the bright side, the NBP reduced children's mental health problems and affected three of the five putative mediators in the expected direction—mother-child relationship quality, effective discipline, and children's experience of divorce-related stressors. And, mediation analyses showed that the program-induced improvements in relationship quality accounted for changes in children's mental health problems, supporting this part of our small theory. Further, the leaders implemented the program with exceptional fidelity, providing confidence in our training and supervision processes. Leaders also endorsed the importance of parents using the skills and they enjoyed running the groups. Importantly, mothers felt very positive about the program (see Wolchik et al., 1993).

We also learned a lot about parts of the program that did not work as intended and used this information to revise the program. Although an aggregate of divorce stressors decreased, interparental conflict was not affected. Given the impact of interparental conflict on children's mental health problems, we decided to revise the curriculum to focus exclusively on it rather than other divorce stressors. Also, mothers in the NBP reported they were more willing to change visitation schedules (e.g., different night or weekend) than those in the waitlist control but contact with fathers did not increase. The process evaluation showed that the leaders consistently delivered all elements in the session related to this component. However, they reported that mothers often shared "war stories" about their divorce and ex-husbands, which made it difficult to acknowledge the value of their children spending more time with their ex-husbands. Based on these observations, we moved the material for this component to an individual one-on-one session. We also found that the program led to decreases rather than increases in support from non-parental adults. The process evaluation data showed that leaders implemented this session as outlined. However, many mothers had moved fairly recently and did not know their neighbors well enough to have their children spend time with them so did not complete the homework for this session. We decided to drop this component for two reasons. First, reducing this barrier to the homework by encouraging mothers to spend time with neighbors would take time away from other program activities. Second, in the context of the program-induced increase in mother-child relationship quality, the decrease in support from non-parental adults made sense. Because of the improved relationship, children may seek support from their mothers rather than other adults. Further, although the program increased effective discipline, leaders felt that more time was needed for revising and getting feedback on the change plans mothers developed to decrease misbehaviors. Based on this feedback, we added another session on discipline and a brief phone contact with the leader after the second discipline session.

Given the positive findings, we conducted another trial to see if we could replicate the results in a larger sample, examine whether the program effects were maintained over time, and whether program benefits could be bolstered by adding a child coping program. The group program for children was run concurrently with the mother program. It targeted four empirically supported mediators: active coping, avoidant coping, negative appraisals of divorce stressors, and mother-child relationship quality. To increase our success in recruiting, in addition to contacting mothers by phone, we conducted brief home visits to invite mothers into the study. Similar to the first trial, significant program effects were found for mother-child relationship quality and effective discipline. The effects on contact with the father and interparental conflict were non-significant. The program decreased externalizing problems and internalizing problems at post-test; changes in externalizing problems were maintained at the six-month follow-up. These changes were mediated by program-induced improvements in mother-child relationship quality and effective discipline (see Wolchik et al., 2000).

Although children in the mother-plus-child program reported higher knowledge of appropriate ways to cope with divorce stressors than those in the mother-only program, there were no significant differences between the two active programs on any of the other mediators or mental health problems either at post-test or six-month follow-up assessments. At the time, we thought it was plausible that the increase in knowledge might require time to affect change in mental health problems. However, at the six-year follow up, the two active program conditions did not differ significantly on any mental health outcomes. So, we combined the two active groups for analysis and compared this group to the control condition. We found program effects on multiple child problems and competencies at the six-year follow up (see Wolchik et al., 2007).

202 Sharlene A. Wolchik and Irwin N. Sandler

Based on the remarkable effects at the six-year follow up, we were motivated to modify the program to be viable in real-world settings and test its "effectiveness." Given the absence of significant differences between the mother-plus-child program and the mother-only program and strong evidence that program-induced improvements in parenting mediated program effects on child behavior problems, we moved forward with the parent-focused program. This change had the important benefit of reducing costs (e.g., leaders, training, materials), which we felt would increase adoption. We selected family courts as our primary partner because they have access to the population of divorcing and separating parents. We developed collaborations with courts in four Arizona counties. Leaders in community agencies delivered the program under our supervision.

We retained the content in the program tested in the second efficacy trial except we deleted the component on increasing contact with the non-residential parent given our inability to change it despite addressing it in an individual session. To promote fidelity, minimize leader burden, and reduce costs of training and implementation, we changed the format of delivery from manual-assisted to DVD-assisted. We also developed a father version of program, which has the same content as the mother version but uses sex-appropriate skill models and testimonials.

Through a comprehensive process of broadening the program to meet the needs of diverse cultural groups (Gonzales et al., 2006), we learned that prevention scientists, providers with expertise in working with Mexican American (MA) and African American (AA) families, and MA and AA mothers who participated in the NBP felt the topics were culturally appropriate. However, these groups suggested numerous "surface structure" changes, such as including more culturally relevant examples, broadening some activities to include extended family members, and including diverse actors in the skills videos. To make the program appropriate for families with children older and younger than those in the efficacy trials (i.e., 8 to 15; 9 to 12) we included discussions of how the activities differ across developmental levels and added tips for using the skills with children across a broad age range. To increase the ease and effectiveness of recruitment, we showed a short video in the brief, information programs that are mandated for divorcing parents in Arizona. Given our goals of getting leaders to a place where they could deliver the program independently and reducing the costs of training and supervision, we modified our methods. The weekly group training was replaced with an asynchronous online training program. Also, instead of participating in weekly supervision of all groups, if leaders demonstrated high fidelity and quality of delivery in their first group, they received minimal supervision for subsequent groups. If not, they continued to receive weekly supervision.

We tested the effects of the revised program in a large-scale effectiveness trial that included ethnically diverse divorcing and separating mothers and fathers. The comparison condition was a two-session program in which parents learned about the same putative mediators but did not practice the skills nor complete home practice. Compared to the comparison condition, the NBP led to higher quality of parenting at post-test and the 10-month follow up and to fewer child mental health problems at the 10-month follow up. The program effects on child mental health were moderated by ethnicity; whereas the effects were significant for non-Hispanic white children, they were not for Hispanic children (see Sandler et al., 2019). However, the analysis that used propensity score matching to compare those in the NBP to a comparable group of families that did not receive any intervention showed that children in Hispanic families in the NBP had significantly lower child mental health problems compared to Hispanics families that received no intervention (Tein et al., 2018).

We learned several important things from this trial. First, the NBP worked for fathers. Second, the NBP was effectively delivered as a service in community agencies. Third, we need to understand why Hispanic families showed benefits from the NBP when compared to those who did not receive any intervention but not when compared with the active control group. Fourth, although showing the invitational DVD in the mandated classes was much easier and less costly than the recruitment methods we previously used, enrolment was still low. Of the 45% of parents who expressed interest in participating, only 20% enrolled in the program, and of those who enrolled, 24% of mothers and 15% of fathers did *not* attend a single session. The low rate of enrolment when the NBP was offered as a free program raised significant concerns about its viability in real-world settings.

Given our commitment to having a population-level impact, we decided to adapt the group-based NBP into a web-based version, which would not only minimize barriers to enrolment but also significantly reduce costs. Using SBIR funding, we adapted the NBP into a web-based program that includes didactic components, skills demonstrations, and interactive exercises. To promote use of the skills with the children, parents are expected to practice the skills and are provided with help to find solutions to difficulties they experience.

Disseminating the NBP

We developed an LLC, Family Transitions: Programs that Work, to disseminate the NBP. Because the development and evaluation of the NBP were funded by grants through the Arizona State University (ASU), the university owns the intellectual property of the program. Our LLC licenses the program back from ASU; ASU receives royalties from sales of the program. Although we have not aggressively marketed the group program, we have contracts with agencies in three states to implement the program in collaboration with referrals from family courts. We plan to market the group- and web-based programs through our LLC. In addition, we will market the web-based program directly to divorced and separated parents and through partnerships with organizations, such as family courts, professional organizations, insurance companies, and providers of non-competing services for divorced and separating families.

Lessons Learned

In our work on the NBP, we learned several things that we think may be helpful for others who are interested in developing preventive interventions. First and foremost, we found the small-theory approach to be extremely valuable. Using research on the potentially modifiable correlates of children's post-divorce adjustment to articulate the processes through which we expected change to occur increased our chances of promoting positive change in children's outcomes. Second, the use of thorough process evaluation and outcome assessments allowed us to identify components of our program that worked as planned, those that did not work as intended, and those that could be improved. Third, mediational analyses were helpful in identifying key ingredients of the program that accounted for change and, thus, need to be preserved in future adaptations for positive program effects to occur. Fourth, our long-term follow ups provided valuable information about the lagged and cascading effects of the program.

As we developed the NBP, we carefully followed the phases outlined in the Prevention Research Cycle (Institute of Medicine, 1994): (1) Identification of the problem; (2) Review of relevant information on risk and protective factors; (3) Development of the program and implementation of pilot and efficacy studies; (4) Conduct of large-scale effectiveness trials; and (5) Implementation and ongoing evaluation in community settings. Since then, alternative methods of program development, such as user-centered design and deployment approaches, have replaced this careful, sequential approach. In these methods, consumers at multiple levels, including the end-consumer and stakeholders in institutions interested in providing the intervention, are heavily involved in designing the program. Further, sustainability strategies are incorporated into the program design from the very beginning. Were we to have started our work on the NBP today rather than nearly 40 years ago, we would have integrated input from multiple consumer groups, such as parents, providers, mental health agency directors, and judges throughout the process of program design. We believe that this type of collaboration is critical for increasing the uptake and public health impact of interventions such as the NBP.

References

Forehand, R., & McMahon, R. J. (1981). *Helping the noncompliant child: A clinician's guide to parent teaching.* New York: Guilford.

Gonzales, N., Wolchik, S., Sandler, I., Winslow, E., Martinez, C., & Cooley, M. (2006, May). *Integrating cultural knowledge with quality management methods to adapt interventions for cultural diversity*. Presented at the Annual Meeting of the Society for Prevention Research, San Antonio, TX

Guerney, L. F. (1978). *Parenting: A skills training manual* (3rd ed.). State College, PA: Institute of the Development of Emotional and Life Skills.

Institute of Medicine. (1994). *Reducing risks for mental disorders: Frontiers for preventive intervention research*. Washington, DC: National Academy Press.

Marlatt, G. A., & Gordon, J. R. (1985). *Relapse prevention: Maintenance strategies in the treatment of addictive behaviors*. New York: Guilford Press.

Novaco, R. A. (1975). *Anger control: The development and evaluation of an experimental treatment*. Lexington, MA: D.C. Heath.

Patterson, G. R. (1975). *Families: Applications of social learning to family life*. Champaign, IL: Research Press.

Pedro-Carroll, J. L., & Cowen, E. L. (1985). The Children of Divorce Intervention Program: An investigation of the efficacy of a school-based prevention program. *Journal of Consulting and Clinical Psychology*, *53*(5), 603–611.

Sandler, I., Wolchik, S., Mazza, G., Gunn, H., Tein, J. Y., Berkel, C., … Porter, M. (2020). Randomized effectiveness trial of the New Beginnings Program for divorced families with children and adolescents. *Journal of Clinical Child and Adolescent Psychology*, *49*, 60–78.

Stolberg, A. L., & Garrison, K. M. (1985). Evaluating a primary prevention program for children of divorce. *American Journal of Community Psychology*, *13*, 1110–1124.

Tein, J.-Y., Mazza, G. L., Gunn, H. J., Kim, H., Stuart, E. A., Sandler, I. N., & Wolchik, S. A. (2018). Propensity score approach to evaluating an effectiveness trial of the new beginnings program. *Evaluation and the Health Professions*, *41*(2), 290–320.

Wolchik, S., Sandler, I. N. Weiss, L., & Winslow, E. (2007). New Beginnings: An empirically based intervention program for divorced mothers to promote resilience in their children. In J. M. Briesmeister & C. E. Schaefer (Eds), *Handbook of parent training: Helping parents prevent and solve problem behaviors*. (pp. 25–62). Hoboken, N.J.: John Wiley & Sons.

Wolchik, S. A., West, S. G., Sandler, I. N., Tein, J.-Y., Coatsworth, D., Lengua, L., … Griffin, W. A. (2000). An experimental evaluation of theory-based mother and mother-child programs for children of divorce. *Journal of Consulting and Clinical Psychology*, *68*(5), 843–856.

Wolchik, S. A., West, S. G., Westover, S., Sandler, I. N., Martin, A., Lustig, J., … Fisher, J. (1993). The children of divorce parenting intervention: Outcome evaluation of an empirically based program. *American Journal of Community Psychology*, *21*(3), 293–331.

Chapter 14

Treatment Foster Care Oregon
Developing an Alternative to Congregate Care

Patricia Chamberlain

Starting Point: Context and Inspirations

The ideas behind the development of the Treatment Foster Care Oregon (formerly known as Multidimensional Treatment Foster Care) model came from the previous work of Gerald Patterson and John Reid on their Social Learning Theory-based parenting interventions and from longitudinal studies conducted in the US and Europe that examined the developmental life course of youth who experienced serious delinquency and antisocial behavior as teenagers. The Social Learning based parenting interventions focused on helping key adults in the child's life to reinforce pro-social, positive behaviors and to apply sanctions when the child misbehaved, broke rules, or did not comply with norms (Patterson & Reid, 1970). Longitudinal studies on the development of delinquency identified the importance of supervision and monitoring of youth whereabouts and associations, prevention of association with delinquent peers, provision of adult mentoring, and positive reinforcement for adaptive normative behaviors (West & Farrington, 1973).

In the early 1980s when I started developing the TFCO model, teenagers who had repeated contacts with the juvenile justice system and who were considered a risk to the safety of the community were placed in residential or group care settings. This practice unfortunately remains a prominent modality today. The essential problem with this practice is that it plays directly into one of the well-documented drivers of the development of delinquency: aggregation of youth with problems with antisocial and delinquent behaviors (Elliott, Ageton, & Huizinga, 1982). Seminal work by Delbert Elliott showed that absent the association of the influence of delinquent peers, the probability of the escalation of delinquency was near zero. The vast majority of teenagers do not commit crimes alone. Delinquency is a team sport. Complementing and adding to that seminal research, Tom Dishion's work on peer contagion identified the specific mechanisms during peer interactions that drove escalations in deviant behavior (e.g., one youth reinforces the others' deviant talk by laughing or otherwise indicating approval; Dishion et al., 1996). Taken together, this work highlighted what a very bad idea it is to house youths together if you are attempting to prevent or reduce the probability of escalating antisocial behavior and delinquency.

Patterson and Reid had demonstrated the power of teaching parents to systematically shape child behavior through their precise responses to that behavior, both positive (using reinforcement) and negative (using limit setting; Patterson et al., 1975).

At the time that I was envisioning the development of the TFCO model I was fortunate to be working as a family therapist at the Oregon Social Learning Center. My mentor was John Reid, who had co-developed the Social Learning Parent Management model with Patterson. John was a talented clinician, a creative thinker, and extraordinarily generous with his time and ideas. John, with Patterson, had developed a home observation coding system designed to quantify family interactions in real time (Reid, 1982). This methodology led to critical insights in the ways that parents and children shaped each other's behaviors over time through their routine daily interactions. For example, observation data clearly showed that when children non-complied or whined and the parents abandoned their requests or gave in to the whining, the probability of non-compliance/whining increased during the next unit of observation time. This work highlighted both the power and the importance of adult reactions to youth behavior, which became a central tenet in the TFCO model.

Strategy and Theory of Change: Early Development of TFCO Model Components

I developed the first version of the TFCO model in response to a Request for Applications from the Oregon Youth Authority (OYA) for program development to create community-based alternatives to incarceration and placements in residential and group care settings. The OYA was concerned about the increasing number of youth housed in institutional or group care settings and was observing high recidivism rates leading to involvement in the adult corrections system in the state.

In designing the model, the two seminal ideas were to (a) extend the Patterson/Reid parenting management Social Learning based parent training models, and (b) to incorporate the knowledge gained from the research led by Elliott & Dishion on the negative effects of delinquent peer association. I applied to OYA and was funded to develop a program for five boys. The boys had been designated by the state to be placed in out-of-home care due to severe and persistent delinquency. The goal of the placement was to protect the community from further crimes and to rehabilitate the boys so that they could be returned to live with family and would not reoffend post placement.

With this context in mind, I designed the basic TFCO model to place one youth in a well-trained and supervised foster home. Once we determined the placement setting that we thought would be optimal for achieving OYA's goals, we worked to develop methods for the surrounding program components, including: (a) close supervision of youth 24/7 and prevention of association with peers with like problems; (b) reinforcement of positive and normative youth behaviors; (c) setting of clear rules and expectations for daily behavior, including the character of daily interactions between the youth and others in the foster home and at school; (d) specification of non-harsh consequences that the foster parents could readily enact in the event of rule violations, problem behavior, or negative interactions; (e) specification of a clear strategy for foster parents to provide youth with mentoring; (f) methods to help youth build skills to interact with non-delinquent peers and succeed in community contexts such as school, sports teams, or interest groups/clubs; and (g) prepare the youth's family for their eventual return home. The OYA contract allowed for a six-month placement, so that created the timeline for accomplishment of the program goals.

The first major barrier that my team and I encountered was recruiting willing community families to provide placements. Foster home recruitment remains a difficult aspect of implementing TFCO today. We have learned much from the creativity of our national and international TFCO sites (now over 100) about recruitment strategies. We also know that recruiting the first cohort of families is the hardest; once the program is up and running, recruitment becomes easier. After numerous community presentations and contacts with service groups, we did recruit five families, one of which was a police officer and his family, who remained foster carers with TFCO for over 20 years. That original family helped us to recruit subsequent families and to expand the capacity of the program; we now recommend paying existing TFCO foster families a "finder's fee" if they refer foster parents who provide placements for TFCO.

Creating Content

The first task at hand was to operationalize the program components listed above while incorporating Patterson and Reid's Social Learning practices. Those practices emphasized teaching through positive reinforcement and setting limits in the instance of minor problems to ideally prevent escalation of negative behaviors. A core program value early on was that close consultation, training, and support of the foster parents was the cornerstone of the model. One of the first considerations was: *how would we prepare and support foster parents to supervise, reinforce, set limits, mentor, and skill build?* Table 14.1 shows an outline of topics covered in the pre-service foster parent orientation, which consisted of six four-hour sessions delivered over a two-week period. After 24 hours of pre-service orientation, foster parents were certified by the state.

Another early consideration was to determine *how to staff the treatment team and conceptualize their roles.* The overarching goals were to provide intensive support to the foster families, to provide the youth with skills, treatment, and reinforcement for normative and positive behavior, and to work with the

Table 14.1 Foster Parent TFCO Orientation Topics

Session #	Topics	Description
1	Orientation and Model Overview	Introduce group members and trainers; describe household, experiences with kids & fostering (if any).
		Overview of treatment components and discussion of the importance of the role of foster families in the treatment team.
		Program supervisor (PS) is the "go to" person, available 24/7,
		Catching problems when they are small; if you think of calling the PS—call!
		Home practice: List five things they like best about teens and five aspects of their parenting they feel good about.
2	Encouraging Cooperation / Adult Requests. Tracking	Review home practice assignment.
		What are reasonable expectations? Definition of cooperation. Spotting small problem behaviors (not minding) and rationale for intervening even though it is a "little" thing.
		How adult requests can be framed, and common pitfalls.
		Home practice: Delivering and watching the reaction to 10 requests with a teen or child you know.
3	Basics of Behavioral Contracting / Tracking Parent Daily Report (PDR)	Review of home practice assignment.
		Discussion of systematic tracking and breaking tasks down in to small steps.
		Using steps toward the target behavior to set-up a point and level system.
		Focusing on the pro-social opposite of problems.
		Discussion of PDR and role play: a five-minute call.
		Home practice: Tracking a target behavior and devising a point and level system to reinforce pro-social opposite behaviors
4	Daily Behavior Management plans using the Point and Level System	Review of home practice assignment.
		Group discussion and review of common problems and pro-social opposites.
		Strategies for dealing with covert problems (stealing, lying).
		Discussion about the use of behavioral incentives.
		Home practice: Identify acceptable daily incentives, identify bonus incentives, schedule for typical school day, schedule for a typical weekend day.
5	Presenting Behavioral Change plans to boys Interacting with Schools	Review of home practice assignment.
		Discussion about how to frame the point and level system so that it will be received positively—role play giving and taking points.
		Daily review: framing it positively, sympathy for point loss.
		School cards: how they work and common pitfalls.
		Home practice: To present the point and level system to the girl and implement.

(Continued)

Table 14.1 (Continued) Foster Parent TFCO Orientation Topics

Session #	Topics	Description
6	Limit Setting	Review of home practice assignment.
		Discussion of the balance between encouragement and limit setting.
		Presentation of the principles of effective non-harsh discipline.
		Role play of time out and privileged removal.
		Strategies to prevent escalation of negative interactions.
		Home practice: To continue to refine and implement the point and level system.

youth's family to prepare them for home visits and for the youth's eventual return home. We needed to have a communication plan for regular contact with the youth's parole/probation officer. We decided that there should be a lead person to coordinate all aspects of the youth's placement, including providing supervision to the youth. Program supervisors (PS) have small caseloads (a maximum of 10 families each). They maintain daily contact with TFCO parents through five-minute PDR calls to collect data on youth problem behaviors and the daily behavior management plan (described below). The role was designed so the PS would not only be the "go to" person for the foster parents, but would supervise the therapists and other members of the treatment team, be the liaison to involved agencies such as the court, parole/probation and the schools, and coordinate all aspects of the youth and family treatment. The role of the family therapist was to meet weekly with biological parents or other aftercare resource. The youth therapist met weekly with the boy. The PS worked to ensure that all of the interventions in the TFCO model (i.e., in the foster home, with the biological or adoptive/relative parents, with the youth, in school) were well synchronized and coherent. Our initial conceptualization of the staff roles is shown in Figure 14.1.

We used this staffing structure for the first year. As we gained experience working with more youth, we realized that there would be a benefit in having a staff member dedicated to coaching and supporting the youth to learn new skills and to serve as a role model. We added the skills coach position. This was needed because the youth individual therapist role focused on treatment of problems with anger management, substance use, and effects of trauma. We felt that teaching youth skills could best be done in community (versus therapy) settings. The skills coach role was developed to meet two objectives: (1) to teach skills that enable youth to solve problems and engage in everyday pro-social interactions, and (2) to engage and integrate youth into pro-social, developmentally appropriate activities. Skills coaches were typically college

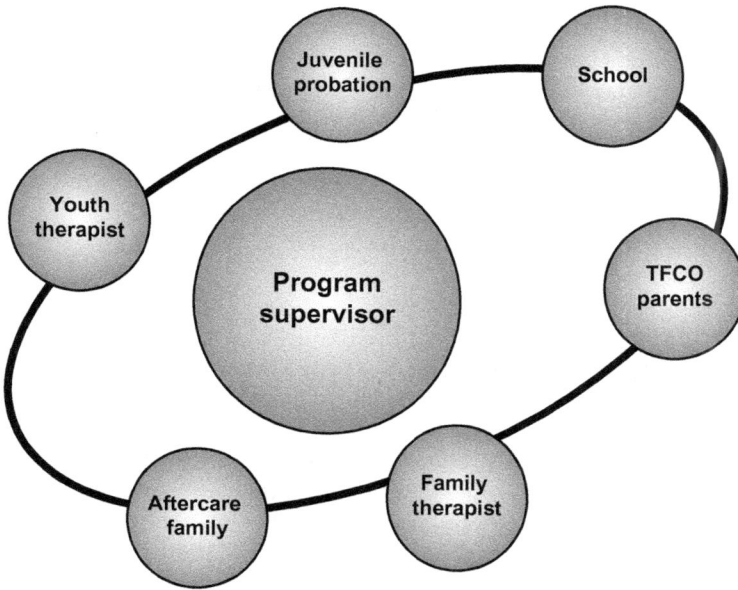

Figure 14.1 Initial Conceptualization of TFCO Staff Roles

students or recent graduates who met one-on-one with the youth weekly. Their job was to provide a consistent, reinforcing environment in which the youth can learn and practice pro-social behavior, problem solving, and coping skills. This was accomplished through one-on-one interactions in the community in which coaches:

- Orient youth toward socially acceptable activities in the community;
- Help youth meet treatment objectives by providing opportunities for skill practice; and
- Provide youth with frequent feedback in a natural (community) environment.

Under the direction of the program supervisor, the skills coach worked with the youth in identified settings to teach, practice, and reinforce appropriate pro-social behavior. Coaches teach by "doing"—and not by talking about what to do. It is not the coach's role to set limits or give consequences, as this could interfere with the role of supportive coach. Progress and problems that occurred in the coaching sessions were reported to the PS. The addition of the coach is an example of one of the many modifications to the model that have been made over the years.

Daily Behavior Management Strategies

As described above, we placed a high value on teaching and supporting youth through the use of frequent reinforcement for normative and adaptive behavior and use of non-harsh clear "light touch" consequences for rule violations and problem behaviors and attitudes. It became obvious early on that it was critical that we devise a system that foster parents could use to enact these strategies on a routine, frequent, daily basis. We wanted the system to focus on easy to apply *standardized* methods for foster parents to facilitate youth positive behaviors and adjustment in the foster home. We needed a method that could be used by foster parents to:

*   Make expectations clear;
*   Encourage and reinforce positive and normative behavior; and
*   Discourage and manage negative behaviour without escalating it.

To do this, we devised a daily behavior management Point and Level System. Table 14.2 shows how the system and rationale were introduced to foster parents. We provided examples of using the system as shown in Table 14.3.

An advantage of placing only one youth per home was that it allowed for the opportunity to individualize the program and specifically the Point and Level system to fit the needs of each youth. Throughout the treatment process for each youth, we worked to consider what specific behaviors we wanted to change or improve. The PS and other clinical staff worked with the foster parents to identify problems in a specific and clear way. For example, if the behavior was something difficult to define or track such as having a negative or angry attitude, we talked with foster parents about instances when they saw or felt the problem happening. Then, we identified the wanted positive opposite behaviors. For example, depending on the youth, to encourage a positive attitude, we might target behaviors to reinforce with points, such as speaking in a friendly tone, helping without being asked, and/or interacting in a kind way with others.

Refining, Expanding, Disseminating

Once TFCO was up and running, we were approached by state leaders in the mental health community. They had difficulty discharging children and teens placed in the state hospital for severe mental illness back into community settings. The Administration for Children and Families, Children's Bureau funded an adaptation of the model in the form of a small randomized controlled trial (RCT) for 9 to18 year olds leaving the Oregon State Hospital; the youth were randomized to TFCO or community discharge as usual (Chamberlain & Reid, 1991). This required an adaptation of the model to fit the needs

Table 14.2 Description for Foster Parents of TFCO Behavior Management Point and Level System

---

Overview and Benefits of the Point and Level System
The Point and Level System is a daily behavior management program. The program specifies the daily activities and behaviors expected, and assigns a number of points the youth can earn for satisfactory performance. The points are a concrete way for parents to teach appropriate skills, reinforce desired behaviors or attitudes, and provide consequences for problem behavior.
Benefits of the point and level system are:

• You and your child are working with the same expectations and understandings.
• It builds in regular opportunities for you to support and encourage your child.
• Consequences are built in to the program.
• You can let the program do the work – you don't have to constantly decide what to do about behavior problems.
• It takes the power struggle out of situations.
• It deals with things as they occur instead of letting them build up.
• The system can be individualized to fit specific needs and situations.
• Program supervisors are always available to help you stay on track.

Some parents are uncomfortable with rewarding kids for what they are supposed to be doing – they expect that kids should behave appropriately without reward. This may be true for "normal" kids, but studies show that kids with severe problem behaviors respond better to tangible rewards than they do to general approval or disapproval. The studies indicate that the typical things parents do, like praising and lecturing, do not affect children and adolescents with severe behavior problems. They respond much better to tangible rewards and consequences.
In the point and level system, the tangible rewards and consequences are distributed through a system of points earned and lost. The youngsters earn points for cooperating and participating in everyday tasks – which is something that many of these kids have not learned to do yet. Throughout the day, they can earn points for expected activities and lose points for breaking rules, including small things such as not listening to an adult or having a surly attitude. The points earned are used to "buy" privileges.
We will show you how to give and take points effectively. With a point system economy, you can be in the position of simply following the program that everyone agreed to. That position enables you to stay out of power struggles with your child and present yourself as an advocate for your child's success with the program.

---

of this population of children and teens. Examples of modifications were to incorporate psychiatry to address medication related issues, and revising the daily behavior management system for use with younger children, and with children and teens with psychotic disorders.

The Oregon Youth Authority program for youth with delinquency grew with additional funding from OYA to expand and funding to conduct an RCT from the National Institute of Mental Health. During these research studies, we had the opportunity not only to test the efficacy of the model but also to

Table 14.3 Example of TFCO Behavior Management Point and Level System for Scott

Example 1: Scott

Scott is 14 and has been in your home for one week. He is pleasant and has been doing a nice job adjusting to your family. Scott likes to please and has been working hard to do what you have asked him in a timely manner and seems willing to volunteer without being prompted.

This morning Scott got up 10 minutes late, dressed, made his bed, and showered. He came to breakfast cheerfully but seemed a bit scattered. After Scott left for school you noticed that he forgot to grab a school card and that the bathroom was messy. His towel and washcloth were left out and he didn't pick up his night clothes. Scott called from school and asked for help because he forgot to take his school card. He had already made a school card on his own for that day and you reassured him that you would talk to the school and give your OK for them to use his home-made card. Scott has seven classes at school. Scott came home from school, put his things away and reported that he was tired. His school card was signed, indicating he attended all his classes with no problems. He did his homework and helped you with dinner. He was a little grumpy before dinner with the other children but turned things around quickly and went to bed on time. See the Point Card for Scott below.

Behavior	Points Available	Adjustments	Points Earned
Up on Time	10	-5	5
Ready in Morning	10	+3 for coming to breakfast cheerfully	11
		-2 for forgetting his school card	
Morning Clean Up	10	-4 for messy bathroom	6
Go to School	5		5
Carry School Card	1/class		7
School Card Bonus	5		5
Behavior in Class	2/class		14
Read and Study	20		20
Chore	10		10
Attitude/Maturity	15 AM	+2 for calling about the school	22
	15 PM	card	22
		+5 for maturity and good decision to call	
		+5 for doing things after school even though he didn't feel well	
		-4 for being grumpy	
		+6 for turning things around and ending day positively	
Volunteering	2–10		0
Extra Chore	5–10		0
Bed on Time	10		10
Total for day = 137			

develop fidelity measures, and investigate what treatment components within the model drove positive outcomes (Eddy & Chamberlain, 2000).

Expanding the Treatment Model to Include Females and to Target Health-risking Sexual Behavior (HRSB)

The next major focus was on adapting the model to address the specific needs of girls with delinquency. Our preliminary work highlighted some overlapping precursors among males and females with serious delinquency and some unique factors specific to girls. For example, for girls the number of parental transitions (i.e., how many times their parenting figure had changed), the girl's lower IQ, and her biological parents' criminality significantly predicted the age of first arrest. Girls' younger age at first arrest was also related to subsequent increased participation in high-risk sexual behavior (HRSB) and increased self-reported delinquency, suggesting that an early first arrest increases the likelihood of cascading risky behaviors, thus increasing the likelihood of poor long-term adjustment. During subsequent years (from 1998 to 2010), in collaboration with Leslie Leve, I modified and tested the model to address the unique clinical needs of girls. In our first study, although preliminary outcomes suggested that there were positive effects associated with participation in TFCO for girls (compared to controls), there were indications that problem patterns remained that were likely to undermine their long-term adjustment. The TFCO intervention did not specifically target reduction of health-risking sexual behaviors (HRSB), and we did not find a differential reduction in HRSBs between TFCO and Group Care (control group) females.

Our analyses showed that engagement in health-risking sexual behavior was related to girls' concurrent self-reports of contraction of a sexually transmitted infection at 12-month follow-up. These results suggested that we could improve the long-term health outcomes for females if we could reduce their engagement in HRSB. We believed that the TFCO intervention effects could be bolstered by a specific intervention component that targeted participation in HRSBs. Specifically, in our next study, we focused on three domains: decreasing substance use, forming and maintaining positive relationships with female peers, and increased knowledge of and comfort in discussing safe sex practices. Subsequent research provided confirmation that these adaptations improved long-term outcomes for females (Leve, Chamberlain, & Reid, 2005; Chamberlain, Leve, & DeGarmo, 2007; Kerr, Leve, & Chamberlain, 2009).

Dissemination

Up until 2000, we had not seriously considered the question of what it would take to disseminate the TFCO model with fidelity, and this remains a major focus of our current work. As we published papers on the model outcomes and presented at conferences, demands for implementation increased. The formal dissemination efforts began with our engagement in the Blueprints for Violence Prevention initiative led by the Office of Juvenile Justice and Delinquency Prevention. We responded to the invitation to become a Blueprint program by writing detailed descriptions of the treatment model and developing fidelity criteria. We had no formal training protocols and initially the training was primarily didactic. We soon discovered that even detailed treatment manuals were not sufficient to transmit the know-how to conduct a successful TFCO program. Throughout the years, our training has become increasingly interactive, and real-time coaching of clinical team members is a critical process for the professional development of TFCO program supervisors and therapists.

Over time, we developed a standardized, yet adaptable, strategy for implementing the model. In 2005 I was funded by NIMH to randomize 51 counties in California and Ohio to one of two strategies for implementing TFCO: either using Community Development Teams where multiple counties implemented together as a cohort, or individual county implementation (the "as usual" condition). As part of that study, in collaboration with Hendricks Brown, I developed the Stages of Implementation Completion (SIC) that allowed for measuring progress on implementation of TFCO. The SIC measures specific activity completion within each of three stages of implementation (pre-implementation, implementation, and sustainment). Having data from this measure allowed us to do research on what it takes to successfully implement the model. The SIC line of research has been expanded by Lisa Saldana and now covers implementation processes and outcomes for over 40 additional EBPs and research-based practices (Nadeem et al., 2018; Palinkas, Campbell, & Saldana, 2018).

At about that time I realized that it was not possible for me to continue to do research and to lead all of the TFCO implementations; something had to give as the requests from potential TFCO sites continued to grow. Additionally, there was a clear need to employ additional staff to be TFCO trainers and to have those people professionally supervised, and the implementations professionally administrated. With John Reid and Gerrard Bouwman (an administrative specialist), I established a separate company (TFC Consultants, Inc.) This company owns the intellectual property for the TFCO model and does all of the implementations, which now number over 100 sites in the US and internationally (www.tfcoregon.com)

Lessons Learned

Intervention development is a team sport. I have had the opportunity to collaborate with trusted and talented colleagues throughout my career. Intervention development is a complex undertaking that requires a range of skills and a high level of persistence. At the outset it might seem like an identified population with specific needs, a solid theory, and clinical acumen is all that it takes to develop an effective, relevant intervention. However, the more the intervention is used, adapted for new populations, and implemented in various contexts and cultures, the clearer it becomes that multiple skills sets and per-spectives are needed to carry it off. Critical to my work have been research colleagues, project managers, methodologists, clinical colleagues, administra-tive specialists, writing partners, public system leaders, psychiatrists, anthro-pologists, social workers, and others. In addition to their needed specialities, the emotional support of trusted colleagues is vital to maintaining optimism through funding and other setbacks and to building a sustainable intervention development and implementation infrastructure. Besides, I have found that it is a lot more fun and gratifying to work in a team than going solo.

Intervention development is iterative. As important as it is to clearly specify model components, it is equally important to modify and add components as imple-mentation experience and the data indicate. In our case, what started as a five-bed experimental alternative to residential/group care for boys with delinquency has become an intervention model used in the mental health, child welfare, and juvenile justice systems in the US and internationally. In a step-by-step fashion, we expanded and/or modified the model to address wider populations of children and teenagers who could benefit from an alternative to residential care. We made cultural adaptations as indicated. We now think of pre-implementation processes as including "Discovery." That is, in any new implementation, we discover as much as we can about the prospective site, and learn about their working pro-cesses and programs. Knowing this allows us to map more easily onto their exist-ing practices and to ease the TFCO program into their organizational culture.

Implementation is more complicated and taxing than intervention development. If you succeed in developing an intervention that fulfils a need and has proven outcomes that sustain, buckle your seatbelt. Understanding how the interven-tion "fits" with existing practices and the extent to which system level changes are needed is critical. For example, the TFCO model requires that foster par-ents have 24/7 on call access to the PS or other program staff. This type of availability is often not an existing feature of programs. I continue to learn and be challenged with every new implementation project.

Continuing directions. After years of working on developing and expanding TFCO, I realized that parts of that model might benefit regular state-supported foster parents. Specifically, the elements of TFCO that focus on supporting and sharpening the skills of foster parents are now offered in KEEP, a model that includes weekly foster and kinship parent groups and weekly Parent Daily Report calls. KEEP has been implemented in all five New York City boroughs, state-wide in Tennessee, in the UK, and in Denmark. Current efforts are to implement state-wide in Oregon (www.keepfostering.org). The fun continues…

References

Chamberlain, P., Leve, L. D., & DeGarmo, D. S. (2007). Multidimensional treatment foster care for girls in the juvenile justice system: 2-year follow-up of a randomized clinical trial. *Journal of Consulting and Clinical Psychology, 75*(1), 187–193.

Chamberlain, P., & Reid, J. B. (1991). Using a specialized foster care community treatment model for children and adolescents leaving the state mental hospital. *Journal of Community Psychology*, *19*(3), 266–276.

Dishion, T. J., Spracklen, K. M., Andrews, D. W., & Patterson, G. R. (1996). Deviancy training in male adolescent friendships. *Behavior Therapy*, *27*(3), 373–390.

Eddy, J. M., & Chamberlain, P. (2000). Family management and deviant peer association as mediators of the impact of treatment condition on youth antisocial behavior. *Journal of Consulting and Clinical Psychology*, *68*(5), 857–863.

Elliott, D. S., Ageton, S. S., & Huizinga, D. (1982). *Explaining delinquency and drug use*. Boulder, CO: Behavioral Research Institute. Retrieved from ncjrs.gov.

Kerr, D., Leve, L. D., & Chamberlain, P. (2009). Pregnancy rates among juvenile justice girls in two RCTs of multidimensional treatment foster care. *Journal of Consulting and Clinical Psychology*, *77*(3), 588–593.

Leve, L. D., Chamberlain, P., & Reid, J. B. (2005). Intervention outcomes for girls referred from juvenile justice: Effects on delinquency. *Journal of Consulting and Clinical Psychology*, *73*(6), 1181–1185.

Nadeem, E., Saldana, L., Chapman, J., & Schaper, H. (2018). A mixed methods study of the stages of implementation for an evidence-based trauma intervention in schools. *Behavior Therapy*, *49*(4), 509–524. doi: 10.1016/j.beth.2017.12.004

Palinkas, L., Campbell, M., & Saldana, L. (2018). Agency leaders' assessments of feasibility and desirability of implementation of evidence-based practices in youth-serving organizations using the Stages of Implementation Completion. *Frontiers in Public Health*. doi: 10.3389/fpubh.2018.00161

Patterson, G. R., & Reid, J. B. (1970). Reciprocity and coercion: Two facets of social systems. In C. Neuringer & J. L. Michael (Eds.), *Behavior modification in clinical psychology* (pp. 133–177). New York: Appleton-Century-Crofts.

Patterson, G. R., Reid, J. B., Jones, R. R., & Conger, R. E. (1975). *A social learning approach to family intervention: Families with aggressive children* (vol. 1). Eugene, OR: Castalia Publishing Co.

Reid, J. B. (1982). Observer training in naturalistic research. In D. Hartmann (Ed.), *Using observers to study behavior: New directions for methodology of social and behavioral science* (Vol. 14, pp. 37–50). San Francisco, CA: Jossey-Bass.

West, D. J., & Farrington, D. P. (1973). *Who becomes delinquent? Second report of the Cambridge Study in Delinquent Development*. Oxford, England: Crane, Russak.

Part V

Adult

Chapter 15

Building Prevention for the Workplace

An Integral and Process-Oriented Approach

Joel B. Bennett, Brittany D. Linde, G. Shawn Reynolds, and Wayne E. K. Lehman

Hindsight might be 20–20. In providing guidance for how to build a prevention program, the benefit of hindsight will play a role here. Our journey started 20 years ago, and the program described below has been used and disseminated since. Before sharing that journey, we emphasize two things upfront. First, a well-built theoretical foundation and heedful integration of previous research is *essential* for developing a sustainable and efficacious program. Studies suggest that there is no substitute for a grounded theory (Charmaz & Belgrave, 2007) or evidence-informed programming (e.g., Small, Cooney, & O'Connor, 2009). Second, to have an impact on dynamic social systems (and workplaces are just that), it is best to adapt a whole-systems or "integral" approach (Bennett, 2018), as well as to consider process-oriented, iterative, or adaptive trials when planning research (e.g., Bhatt & Mehta 2016).

Our team does not target individual-level risks and behaviors without understanding the system and culture (and subcultures) within which individuals socialize and work. With an attitude of exploration, we adapt program features according to what we learn through our relationship with the system. We assume that unlike treatment, biomedical, and pharmaceutical interventions, *prevention* programs that are sensitive to local social context and social determinants can only work within an integral and process-oriented framework. This is an "inside-out" process that relies greatly on, and empowers, the end-user (cf. Miller, Rubinstein, Howard, Crabtree, 2019). Note that in this chapter, "training" refers to the definition typically used in workplace human resource nomenclature; that is, a structured program delivered to employees with objectives to develop or increase job-related skills and abilities. Also, the terms "trainer" and "facilitator" are used interchangeably to refer to the individual who delivers the curriculum to a group of participating employees.

As prevention interventionists, we are more like diplomat-consultants than medical doctors. We do not administer a pre-fabricated and finished curriculum. Instead, we start with extant and evidence-informed content, process consultation tools, and then work iteratively with stakeholders and the target population to create an adapted program that suits the needs and environment of the client. We still use this "inside-out" process to meet specific client needs.

Starting Point

Research interest in substance use in the workplace grew following the inception of the Drug Free Workplace Act (1988) (e.g., Normand, Lempert, & O'Brien, 1994). The "Workplace Project" at the Institute of Behavioral Research (IBR) at Texas Christian University (TCU) was funded through the National Institute on Drug Abuse's Office of Workplace Initiatives (National Institute on Drug Abuse DA04390 to D. Dwayne Simpson & Wayne E.K. Lehman). Dr. Lehman had worked with municipalities to understand the scope and context of the problem, conducting surveys on municipal employee alcohol and drug use. Dr. Joel Bennett was hired a few years into this project to analyze data and outline a prevention curriculum that could apply to workplaces universally. The municipal workforce was a useful context for developing a universal program because city workers represent a wide variety of job types.

As noted, there had not been much systematic research in the area when we began this line of work, and there was a clear need for evidence-informed training and development for prevention in the working population. As demonstrated in several NIDA monographs on drugs in the workplace (e.g., Gust et al., 1990), research findings were primarily descriptive. Most drug free workplace training back in the 1990s and still today is focused on identifying "signs and symptoms" of employee substance use problems and education about employer policies. Supervisor training, depending on occupation and industry, also includes constructive confrontation and referral to employee assistance programs (EAP). However, the survey data and previous studies in occupational alcoholism (e.g., Roman, 1990; Trice & Sonnenstuhl, 1990) unequivocally pointed to workplace culture and occupational subcultures of drinking ("drinking climate") as strong influences on employee substance use (and health behaviors in general). In the early 1990s, workplaces were still in the early years of implementing Drug Free Workplace (DFWP) guidelines, which often included five elements: (1) a clearly written policy; (2) drug-testing; (3) supervisor training; (4) employee training; and (5) access to counseling and treatment. These guidelines were not explicitly designed to address workplace culture, social context, and the dynamic interchange between culture and guideline adaptation.

Strategy and Theory of Change

Strategies that align with grounded theory are built inductively, driven by data, and ideally draw from previously known principles in the field. Moreover, when dealing with complex systems like workplaces, a sound strategy requires obtaining perspectives from a range of stakeholders and knowledge experts. Hence, our strategy was informed by DFWP standards, existing data from the target population, information provided by local EAP providers ("boots on the ground"), previous scientists, and in our case a team of applied scientists.

Having arrived at the IBR project after employee survey data had already been collected, Dr. Bennett was able to tweak new surveys and explore new hypotheses prior to curriculum development. This gave him the ability to first combine previous interests, and then apply such knowledge to the task of curriculum development. Our work was informed by knowledge at the intersection of several disciplines: Applied social psychology, group dynamics, organizational climate and culture, process consultation, focus group methods, codependency, and family systems models of alcoholism.

In addition, the IBR team worked closely with the surveyed municipalities. City officials were interested in any problems identified in exploratory surveys. As a result of their interest, the IBR team worked with EAP professionals in two municipalities (one internal workplace EAP and one external EAP contractor) and human resources. Gaining their insight about local policies, current implementation of DFWP, and human resource benefits (e.g., access to insurance for treatment) helped us to navigate practical aspects of the project. For example, one HR professional shared information about incidents involving employee drug-testing and how more proactive efforts could have helped an employee who was fired for substance misuse.

Learning from experts in related fields is also important when developing program content. Pioneering researchers in occupational alcoholism, worker drug prevention, and EAP studies were quite influential. This included Dr. Harrison Trice on the role of EAPs in work culture; Dr. William Sonnenstuhl on employee self-referral; Dr. Genevieve Ames on codependence in work; Dr. Judd Allen on healthy work cultures; and Dr. Royer Cook on health promotion as a workplace strategy. Colleagues at the IBR also served as internal consultants, including Norma Bartholomew (curriculum development), Kirk Broome (statistician), George Joe (statistician), and graduate students especially Jamie Forst and Shawn Reynolds.

Based on the above inputs, we applied a grounded theory approach to develop an intervention, rather than build completely from scratch. By "grounded theory" we mean studying the population and previous empirical research on risk and protective factors and, as much as possible, synthesizing perceived needs of the target population and results of research into a model of one's own. One can also borrow from existing theories, especially those that have established viability with meta-analysis or systematic review.

For the initial design of Team Awareness (TA), we applied thinking on protective and risks factors (cf. Durlak, 1998) as located *within the workplace context*, described by over a dozen previously published IBR studies. We then integrated the findings of these papers into an article that proposed the original theory behind TA (Bennett, Lehman, Reynolds, 2000). Figure 15.1 shows the conceptual model that was developed for the 2000 paper, with an understanding that there was an unexplored "black box" of workplace context. This black box idea—borrowed from engineering science—assumes that there is a system which can be viewed in terms of its inputs and outputs, without any

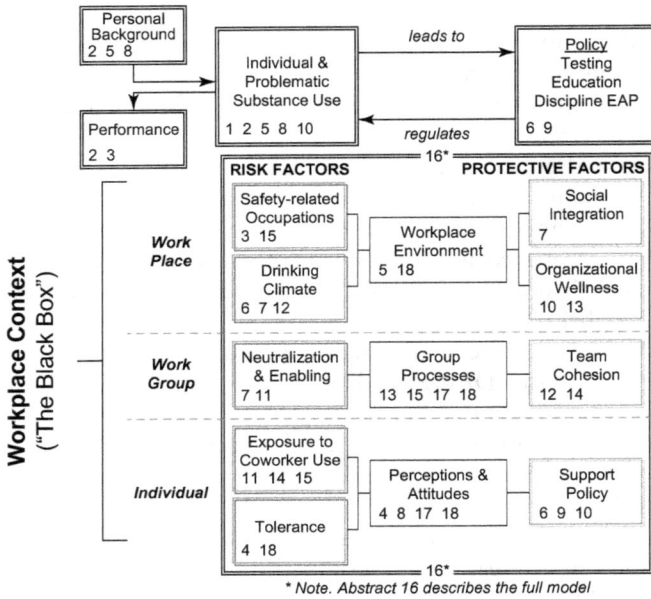

Figure 15.1 The Original Model for Team Awareness, Grounded Theory (1990–2002)

Note: The numbers in the right figure refer to supporting research articles. An online version of these articles and abstracts can be found at https://www.slideshare.net/JoelBennett/team-awaren ess-for-mental-wellbeing-in-the-workplace-original-theoretical-article. (1) Lehman & Simpson, 1990; (2) Lehman & Simpson, 1992; (3) Holcom, Lehman, & Simpson, 1993; (4) Holcom, Lehman & Lord, 1993; (5) Lehman, Farabee, Holcom & Simpson, 1995; (6) Bennett & Lehman, 1996a; (7) Bennett & Lehman,1996b; (8) Forst & Lehman, 1997; (9) Bennett & Lehman, 1997a; (10) Bennett & Lehman, 1997b; (11) Lehman, Farabee & Bennett, 1998; (12) Bennett & Lehman, 1998; (13) Bennett, Lehman & Forst, 1999; (14) Bennett & Lehman, 1999a; (15) Bennett & Lehman, 1999b; (16) Bennett, Lehman & Reynolds, 2000.

knowledge of its internal workings. The figure details elements about these internal workings; i.e., the context informed by specific IBR studies. In the following sections, we describe the grounded theory, the general principles and curriculum as relevant to fidelity, and a summary of subsequent dissemination efforts and adaptations.

Original Model

The figure (top) identifies a core employer assumption that *workers' problematic substance use should be addressed through policy*. Typically, these are DFWPs that prohibit substance use and, ideally, provide education as a preventative measure. However, research indicated that this assumption downplays the *contexts* (e.g., workplace culture, social norms, workplace resources) which significantly influence individual risks and policy implementation. In some situations, workplace policy only serves a symbolic function for the company to "look good." In such situations, supervisors may ignore drinking cultures or other unhealthy social norms among work groups. Moreover, social norms and occupational subcultures develop that tend to ignore or psychologically minimize the risks associated with problem drinking or related counter-productive behaviors. This social "neutralization" of problems (cf. Robinson & Kraatz, 1998) appeared to be a critical risk factor that any effective program should address.

Accordingly, we identified that it was important to build a workplace training that addressed risks and protective factors at three levels: workplace, work group, and individual risks. Details on how the training addresses these three levels are described in the next section. In particular, we considered it essential to focus on peer-to-peer interaction in the work group and give workers tools to proactively support coworkers at risk (as opposed to neutralizing, stigmatizing, ignoring, enabling, or tolerating their risky behavior).

Creating Content Theory and Observation

The targeted behaviors and attitudes targeted by Team Awareness were identified from two sources: the studies and model described above (Figure 15.1), and what we learned through direct conversational input from stakeholders. This section describes how we learned from these inputs. The next section describes many of the actual exercises and tools taught in the training.

We labeled the stakeholder input "Discovery" and utilized key informant interviews, focus groups, and information about mental health and social issues provided by human resources, employee relations, and EAP professionals

At the same time that the IBR team was reviewing the survey data and building the grounded theory, we began an inductive-deductive application of ideas to possible program content. With a theory and ideas for content in hand, we first conducted focus groups with municipal employees, supervisors and EAP and HR professionals. We had general principles about what risk and protective factors were important to address, and then (deductively) created sample slides, discussion items, and activities to showcase or pilot with these employees. For example, we conducted a serial focus group where we met with a group of staff on four separate occasions over a period of six weeks (Bennett et al., 2000). These sessions engaged employees in open discussion and brainstorming about potential training content. We also introduced interactive group exercises, obtained feedback, and made changes to the content. These changes to pilot curriculum were (inductively) made based on input from the end-users.

Several examples of what we learned through this process provide insight into why we determined that group or team-processes and psychological safety were so important and why we should develop a curriculum that centered on creating group experiences and opportunities for employees to share, learn together, and help each other.

- After three focus group sessions, where stories were shared about alcohol and drug use, one participant disclosed that they had been afraid and were in denial that their teenage child was misusing drugs. The safety of the group gave this participant an awareness that was not otherwise available.
- A group of supervisors shared that there was one employee who kept "beating the system." Everyone knew this employee was abusing alcohol at work and the older supervisors would just hand the problem off to the newer supervisors because they had resigned themselves to their belief that nothing they could do would work.
- A group of workers who liked to go out for beers after work revealed that one colleague had an intermittent but sometimes significant drinking problem. They were at a loss as to what to do because they did not want to jeopardize the employment of their colleague.

Such discussions revealed that because of cultural and social climate factors (e.g., alienation, drinking climate) that impact employee substance misuse, the training would need to be highly interactive to insure confidentiality, help participants work through complex scenarios (like those above), encourage some level of participant self-disclosure, and take place across multiple sessions in order to enhance transfer of learning (Broad & Newstrom, 1992). Consequently, guidelines were developed to foster a sense of psychological safety (Edmondson, 1999) within the training environment (i.e., CHAT guidelines: Confidentiality, Honor, Anonymity, and Trust). Because of the team-focus, it was also critical that as many individuals from a work group be present and take the training together. We rarely trained a lone worker who was not also accompanied by another peer and sometimes—if scheduling allowed—we attempted to train entire work groups together. Detail on actual content is described in the next section.

Dr. Lehman had received funding from the National Institute of Drug Abuse (NIDA) to conduct an experimental study utilizing a cluster randomized trial where work groups (within departments) would be randomly assigned to receive the training or be placed in a wait-list control group. A primary consideration was that departments with the highest risk for substance use may be the least willing to participate. One department with relatively high levels of drinking (based on survey data) withdrew from the initial study because (or at least it appeared that) we were getting too close to underlying workplace issues. There were also methodological considerations associated with conducting the experimental study in a way that would reduce contamination from one work group (receiving the training) to another (in control condition).

Creating Content: The How and What

As Figure 15.2 shows, we created content in three steps: (1) from discovery, we identified six different key issues to inform design (based on our previous research, grounded theory, and observations of how stakeholders responded to pilot content); again, curriculum development focused on group processes; (2) we created initial module objectives for the training curriculum; and (3) following these objectives, we either selected or modified slides and activities from our piloting in focus groups within the discovery phase or created new elements based on feedback.

The following paragraphs provide examples of content for the six modules. Two design factors emerged because of the need to address group processes and psychological safety. First, the aforementioned CHAT guidelines around confidentiality were introduced in Module 1 and reiterated throughout all modules, which were successively organized to encourage progressively increased levels of self-disclosure and make it safer for individuals to discuss the six issues identified in the model. We sought to create a climate of compassion such that coworkers could feel comfortable reaching out for help if needed and also talk with others about issues that emerged from discussions.

Second, we wanted to help participants reach the point where they would potentially be motivated and know how to help a coworker, either directly through compassionate listening or by referring them to the EAP. We aimed to help develop workers' peer-referral skills so that they can talk with a colleague if they suspect that a coworker is having personal difficulties (e.g., stress of any type as well as overt signs of substance misuse). We framed the process of helping a co-worker as the NUDGE model: Notice, Understand, Decide, use Guidelines, and Encourage. We built participant understanding of these five components across the sessions, and then introduced the integrated NUDGE in the last module.

Several factors led to the initial idea of this NUDGE model as a capstone. First, the lead author had been trained as a clinical psychologist, and had applied principles of recovery and codependence in group process settings (e.g., Schaef, 1986) and had taught undergraduate courses on group processes (e.g., Egan, 1973). Second, as noted above, the work of Harrison Trice and William Sonnenstuhl on workplace alcohol dynamics indicated the importance of small groups and the social construction of social norms as influencing whether at-risk employees would self-refer for help and/or be open to encouragement from colleagues (e.g., Sonnenstuhl, 1990). Third, Norma Bartholomew had introduced the IBR team to concepts from motivational interviewing (Rollnick & Miller, 1995) and suggested adapting them for workplace use. Finally, the lead author had participated in an ASIST Suicide

CONTENT DERIVATION (1996 – 2002)

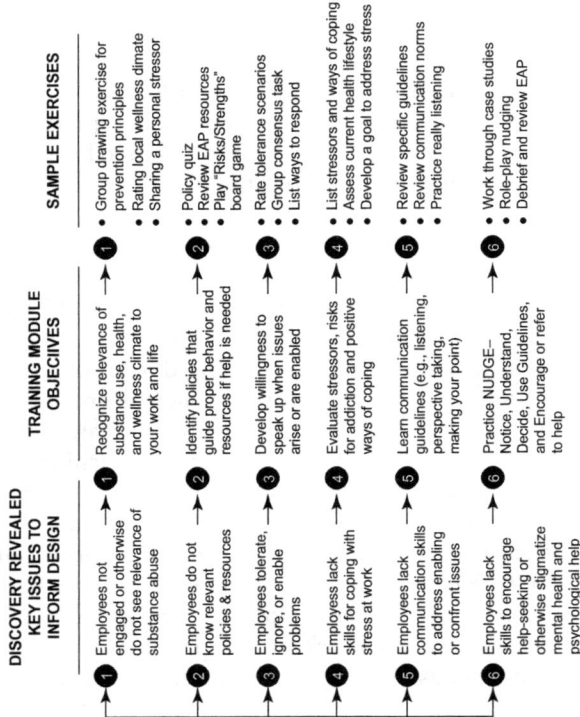

GROUNDED THEORY

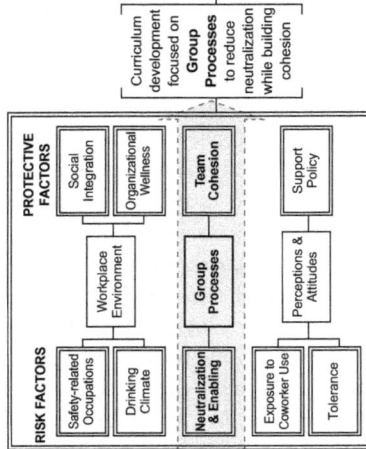

DISCOVERY REVEALED KEY ISSUES TO INFORM DESIGN	TRAINING MODULE OBJECTIVES	SAMPLE EXERCISES
1 Employees not engaged or otherwise do not see relevance of substance abuse	**1** Recognize relevance of substance use, health, and wellness climate to your work and life	• Group drawing exercise for prevention principles • Rating local wellness climate • Sharing a personal stressor
2 Employees do not know relevant policies & resources	**2** Identify policies that guide proper behavior and resources if help is needed	• Policy quiz • Review EAP resources • Play "Risks/Strengths" board game
3 Employees tolerate, ignore, or enable problems	**3** Develop willingness to speak up when issues arise or are enabled	• Rate tolerance scenarios • Group consensus task • List ways to respond
4 Employees lack skills for coping with stress at work	**4** Evaluate stressors, risks for addiction and positive ways of coping	• List stressors and ways of coping • Assess current health lifestyle • Develop a goal to address stress
5 Employees lack communication skills to address enabling or confront issues	**5** Learn communication guidelines (e.g., listening, perspective taking, making your point)	• Review specific guidelines • Review communication norms • Practice really listening
6 Employees lack skills to encourage help-seeking or otherwise stigmatize mental health and psychological help	**6** Practice NUDGE– Notice, Understand, Decide, Use Guidelines, and Encourage or refer to help	• Work through case studies • Role-play nudging • Debrief and review EAP

Curriculum development focused on **Group Processes** to reduce neutralization while building cohesion

RISK FACTORS

Safety-related Occupations

Drinking Climate

Workplace Environment

Neutralization & Enabling

Group Processes

Exposure to Coworker Use

Tolerance

Perceptions & Attitudes

PROTECTIVE FACTORS

Social Integration

Organizational Wellness

Team Cohesion

Support Policy

Figure 15.2 Content Derivation: From Grounded Theory to Sample Exercises

Prevention training (Gould et al., 2013), which used role plays to help "gate-keepers" or "bystanders" develop skills for having a conversation with some-one showing signs or symptoms of suicide.

In order to build the NUDGE model, we introduced an overall framework for prevention and highlighted the importance of substance use for health and work in Module 1. Module 2 reviews general and workplace-specific policies around alcohol and drug use, as well as identifying work group norms around alcohol. In Module 3, participants are supported in speaking up and actively engaging with co-workers around substance use. Module 4 presents alcohol and drug addiction in terms of stress and coping, giving participants a language and conceptual frame for managing their own use as well as supporting others. Module 5 focuses on basic communication skills that participants can use with co-workers who need help. At the same time that we taught these conceptual frameworks and skills throughout the first modules, implementation of the NUDGE model also required the development of trust within a work group. The modules were designed to build trust amongst the participants though increasing levels of sharing and group exercises. We provide more detail on this capstone module (Module 6) following a review of the modules with examples of how content was derived for each.

Module 1—Relevance

The objective of the first module was to recognize the relevance of health, mental health, substance misuse, and wellness climate to your work and life. Several exercises were designed primarily to get participants talking and applying ideas to their own personal situation. This includes an interactive and fun review of seven "ounce of prevention principles" where participants receive a pocket-sized card (see Figure 15.3), brain-storm about images they can associate to each principle, and then one volunteer draws that image on a flip-chart and is applauded (or kindly chided) by the group. These principles orient participants to the rest of the training and are re-iterated in each module. The "group drawing" exercise helps "break the ice" and builds the protective factor of group cohesiveness.

Participants also worked—in pairs and in small groups—on three exercises that are all debriefed. These exercises were more or less developed "from scratch" but used common principles found in many adult learning training programs, like those from the Association for Talent Development (www.atd.org) or the classic text "The Adult Learner" by Malcolm Knowles. These exercises included: (1) A "Big Picture" Sentence Completion task, where participants fill in blanks for sentences asking for perceptions of the level of both "substance use" and "sense of community" at national, state, and local levels, and in their own workplace; (2) A "Team Risks & Strengths" rating exercise where participants confidentially rate items from brief versions of our work climate scales and then the entire group's response is anonymously tabulated,

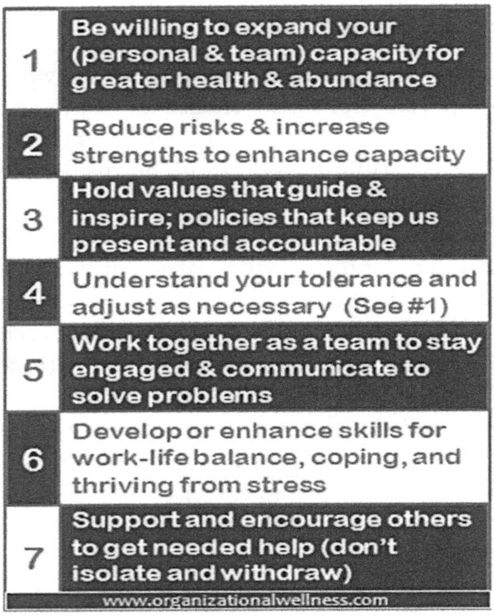

1	Be willing to expand your (personal & team) capacity for greater health & abundance
2	Reduce risks & increase strengths to enhance capacity
3	Hold values that guide & inspire; policies that keep us present and accountable
4	Understand your tolerance and adjust as necessary (See #1)
5	Work together as a team to stay engaged & communicate to solve problems
6	Develop or enhance skills for work-life balance, coping, and thriving from stress
7	Support and encourage others to get needed help (don't isolate and withdraw)

www.organizationalwellness.com

Figure 15.3 Ounce of Prevention Principles (pocket-card handout)

presented back, and discussed; and (3) "Finding Your Voice," a two-person exercise to practice really listening when someone shares a problem or stressor. In turn, these three exercises help to make the issues of substance use and social connection personally relevant, create a concrete experience of the meaning of "work climate" and its importance to personal well-being, and introduce the importance of communication and being able to listen in the face of stress. Overall, the facilitator keeps checking for signs of understanding/interest and directly asks how much the exercises pertain to participant's personal or professional life.

Module 2—Team Ownership of Policy

Objective: Identify policies that guide proper behavior and resources if needed. As described above, the curriculum was partly informed by Drug Free Workplace standards, which includes a review of policies (restrictions on substance use), education on signs and symptoms, as well as knowing where to obtain help if an employee or family members has problems (e.g., EAP, health benefits for treatment). A core idea of this module is that it is always better to proactively seek out and get help/resources as opposed to continue with risky behavior and slip, get hurt, or get caught. This module is also customized to the policies and benefits of the local setting. Specifically, PowerPoint slides review local policies (e.g., types of drug-testing, restrictions for alcohol use, disciplinary procedures) and ways to access help (e.g., telephone number of and services covered by the EAP). Importantly, these ideas are also presented through a team-competitive board game.

The game idea came from a training conference (Association of Training & Development), where the lead author attended sessions on game-based learning. Three to four teams of participants work together to get answers to questions, collect points, and move their game piece on a board that illustrates different risks and strengths depending on whether questions are answered correctly. For example, a risk is "members in your work group believe that getting help for a problem is a sign of weakness" and a strength is "a co-worker tells you he is stressed with a supervisor. You listen and help to solve the problem." The decision to use a highly engaging game was also made because most policy instruction is often dry and unmemorable.

Module 3—Reducing Stigma and Tolerance: Increasing Responsiveness

Objective: Develop a willingness to speak up when issues arise. This module came from several previous studies conducted at the IBR (e.g., Holcom, Lehman, Lord, 1993) where employees were presented with written descriptions of different drug-related scenarios (e.g., a coworker repeatedly comes to work late with a hangover). Employees rated how likely they would tolerate (i.e., do nothing, look the other way) versus respond to the situation. The exercise first requires individuals to work independently to rate their likely response across six to ten scenarios. Then participants assemble into small groups, are instructed to come to consensus on selecting a final rating, and are encouraged to discuss all sides and honor differences of opinion. By this time in the training, because of the CHAT guidelines and a growth in trust, the majority of participants are willing to share their ideas and opinions within these small groups. This module deliberately introduces the concept of "drinking climate" and encourages participants to reflect on the relative risks and benefits of using alcohol as a way to socially bond, relax, or otherwise have leisure time with coworkers.

Module 4—Stress, Problem Solving, and You

Objective: Identify Stressors, risks for addiction, and positive ways of coping. Module 4 helps participants identify lifestyle (wellness) factors that protect from illness and contribute to overall well-being, and explore healthy alternatives to the use of alcohol and drugs whenever possible. Participants self-assess their physical, emotional, and spiritual health and diverse ways of coping. Responses from the group are recorded on flip-charts and signs of stress are identified. This approach uses a cognitive-behavioral model of: (1) Identify the

Stressor; (2) Evaluate How you Process the Stressor; and (3) Select a Coping Response. Module 4 guides participants through this process to help them to select health and wellness goals (that can also mitigate addictive tendencies), as well as encourage self-referral for any health problem (e.g., anxiety, alcohol use) as supported by research on self-referral (Sonnenstuhl, 1982). Module 4 was deemed the "Wellness" module in that it primarily discusses stress, resilience, and well-being and secondarily presents addiction in that context (see Cook, 1985; Cook, Back, Trudeau, 1996).

Module 5—Communication

Objective: Learn communication guidelines (e.g., listening, taking perspective, making your point). Module 5 reviews the importance of effective communication. One of the authors of the training curriculum (Norma Bartholomew) had developed other training manuals for IBR on communication and felt that skills for direct communication and motivational interviewing should also be introduced into the training. Norma's input coincided with what was known about "constructive confrontation" in the workplace alcohol/EAP literature, which presented guidelines for how supervisors should set up a meeting with an employee presenting symptoms of alcohol use disorder (e.g., Trice & Beyer, 1984). A separate module for supervisors was created to help them with their reluctance to have these conversations (Bennett & Lehman, 2002). One of the exercises in this module is a follow-up and deeper dive into the "Really Listening" exercise in Module 1. Again, participants pair up and are given additional guidelines on how to listen (e.g., body language, not interrupting, avoid judgment, etc.).

Module 6—Capstone: NUDGE

Objective: Practice NUDGE—Notice, Understand, Decide, use Guidelines, and Encourage. In early focus groups, we thought to introduce this model via a single role play from a case study in which two participants would act out the peer-to-peer encouragement. We learned from these focus groups that many employee participants were not eager to (and may be embarrassed) to role play in front of their peers, that different role play situations were needed, and that it would be more comfortable for participants to label the activity as a "case study" rather than a role play. As a result, we created several one-page case studies for participants to use as a basis for role plays. This included examples like 'Sam who is the life of the party and tends to drink more' and 'John the athlete who appears to be misusing pain-killers'. Also, as suggested by the sequence of the previous modules, participants found the idea of peer encouragement as a natural next step following learning about responsibility (policy Module 2 and Ounce of Prevention Principle 3), being more responsive than tolerant (Module 3, Principle 4), and knowing how to communicate without offending the person in need of help (Module 5, Principle 5).

The resulting content then first introduces participants to the NUDGE model and explains how it builds upon the previous modules. Then, participants are organized into groups of three individuals: A nudger, a nudgee, and an observer. Each group is provided with the case study of an employee (usually from their own or related occupation) who has some health-related problem, often involving misuse of alcohol, prescription drugs, or an illegal drug. The "nudgee" was instructed to resist being nudged (getting help). The "nudger" was instructed to utilize skills and ideas learned in previous modules (e.g., really listening). The observer was instructed to coach the nudger and also make sure they used collateral such as the EAP handout or other tools to help with the conversation. Each group worked independently and all debriefed the process.

Findings, Adaptations, and Replications

The first output from our research were published studies that focused on process findings—factors that influenced implementation, such as work group and classroom dynamics—as well as outcomes. Initial and later studies found that Team Awareness reduced risks for problem drinking, increased help-seeking (to the EAP), reduced stigma, reduced in drinking climate, and improved supervisor responsiveness to problems, coping, and wellness climate (e.g., Bennett & Lehman, 2001, 2002; Patterson et al., 2005; Petree et al., 2012; Reynolds & Bennett, 2015).

Initial research also examined process-findings that may help identify ways to adjust how the delivery of training could be improved in future implementation. For example, analyses of data from the original clinical trial revealed potential mediators of program outcomes—especially drinking climate and coworker perceptions of stigma (e.g., see Bennett et al., 2004). In addition, we used behavioral coders for each training session to rate worker behaviors, such as level of self-disclosure. Sessions with higher average training satisfaction also had higher levels of participant self-disclosure (Bennett, Reynolds, Lehman, 2003).

Together, these findings produced insights that led to the development of related programs and studies. These programs and studies, created and managed by Dr. Bennett and staff at Organizational Wellness & Learning Systems (OWLS), included training for small businesses (i.e. *Small Business Wellness Initiative*), *Team Resilience* for young workers, *Team Readiness* for the military (US National Guard), and online or e-learning adaptations (e.g., Bennett et al., 2018a). Independent researchers also replicated some intervention findings (e.g., Burnhams et al., 2015; Cadiz et al., 2012). Further, OWLS has consulted with numerous organizations in helping to adapt principles and content from this program. The module on stress (Module 4) has been the most widely adapted, with over 300 individuals trained as trainers (e.g., Bennett et al., 2018b).

Since 2002, several in-depth (often week-long) train-the-trainers in the original TA curriculum have been delivered to prevention specialists and trainers. As a result, TA has been used for different work populations (e.g., Native American Tribal Government workers, African-American ex-offenders, young restaurant workers, electrician apprentices, public health workers, Youth Corp workers). Dr. Bennett has worked with academics and government agencies in several foreign countries (e.g., Gelmi, Vimercati, Celata, 2017; Burnhams et al., 2015). Through extensive consultation with these groups we now view the intervention itself as only one piece of the solution in any social system design, especially amongst working adults.

Guidance Models

We developed two models for guiding or consulting with others in prevention design. First, our current methods for intervention development follows a similar process to the original TCU studies, described above. These methods were first documented in a "research-to-practice" article (Bennett et al., 2010). We use a five-step procedure for either deriving and testing a new intervention or for adapting TA (see Figure 15.4). Second, we created a meta-theory (Bennett, Cook, Pelletier, 2011) that positions this 5-step *intervention* process within a broader context of four dimensions that includes the intervention, capacity building, fidelity, and adaptation itself. We identified these elements from studies that were later incorporated into the Strategic Prevention Framework from the Substance Use and Mental Health Services Administration. These four elements—the intervention, adaptation, fidelity, and capacity building—work together as one integral system to influence program impact.

The basic phases involved in creating or deriving a new prevention program are depicted in Model 1, the left portion of Figure 15.4. The five core features of this process are:

1. **Discover** (assess current state) or understand the needs, risks, protective factors, environments, resources, cultures of the target population.
2. **Adapt** or modify the pre-existing curriculum to address the needs, risks, and strengths identified in discovery; that is, we gather evidence-informed content (e.g., from the studies detailed in Figure 15.1, other previous literature, and from the target population) that can best address the needs and risks identified in the Discover phase. Adapt is the process that we, as consultants, use to reflect to the client that we are adapting content that is based on pre-existing knowledge of what is likely to work *within the client's setting*. In this way, the adapt phase occurs *before* the next design phase because we have to consider client-relevant factors. Material in the *earlier* portions of the adaptation phase is more of an initial showcase, prototype or "proof of concept" and is shown to the client before full design

Model 1
The Process of Deriving and
Testing New (or adapted) Training

Model 2
Integral Model of Prevention
(viewing intervention in context)

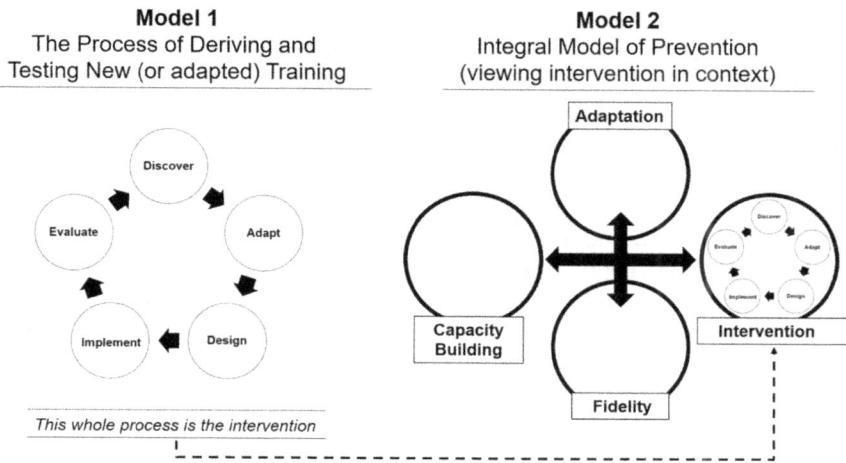

Figure 15.4 Two Models for Intervention Development and Sustainability

takes place to ensure that the client "signs-off" or agrees that the proposed design is relevant, feasible, and supported.

3. **Design** the program, consulting with the target population through any further prototyping, piloting, conducting a feasibility trial, or a "test and learn". We call this "Design" to represent what the client perceives explicitly happens in this step. That is, we are designing the final program elements in preparation for delivery and for the client.

4. **Implement** the program.

5. **Evaluate** outcomes, including those that matter to the target population.

The diagram on the right in Figure 15.4 (Integral Model) situates the five steps of deriving a new intervention inside the sphere labeled "Intervention" (shown to the far right). Intervention development is only one of the four social forces that ultimately impact the long-term success and sustainability of the program in a workplace setting (See Bennett, Cook, Pelletier, 2011). Based on our experience, a curriculum developer who embarks on the five-stage intervention derivation process (left in Figure 15.4) would benefit from initially thinking about all four "big picture" processes (right in Figure 15.4).

These four forces stand in a dynamic relationship to each other with "tension" existing between them. For example, the success of an intervention depends, to some extent, on the time taken to build capacity and readiness (i.e., stakeholder buy-in). In our work, capacity building tends to overlap with the "Discover-Adapt" phase of the five-step procedure. By showing a potential curriculum to stakeholders (e.g., via focus groups) we are asking them to participate in sharing information back-and-forth to others, including the stakeholders they represent. These initial stakeholder groups serve as proxy ambassadors. Tensions between capacity building and intervention do arise at times, especially when time pressures to deliver the program are high due to budget, policy, or other factors. Tensions between capacity building and intervention are relatively lower when, as in our and other's work (e.g., adaptive designs, user-based designs), capacity building is explicitly woven into the process itself.

In a parallel fashion, the local or case-by-case success of an intervention depends on the proper balance between adhering to fidelity versus making customized changes to the original program in order to meet local needs and cultural sensitivity. The tension between fidelity and adaptation is greater when there are mandates surrounding fidelity or there are strict contingencies around scalability. That tension is diminished when the intervention itself seeks to empower end-users as local "owners" of the program (e.g., white labeling, open-source non-exclusive licensing). For example, non-profit grantees are sometimes required to use evidence-based programs for high-risk local populations. These grantees struggle because they need to fulfill the requirements of grantors who may not understand the local needs of the target population. Prevention program developers may make considerable efforts (e.g., clinical trials) to develop very well-informed program designs, but those programs end up on a shelf when local concerns are neglected. For this reason, addressing the other processes (adaptation, capacity building) are as important as developing the program content along with clear guidelines for fidelity.

Fidelity, Dissemination and Sustainability

In designing prevention in the way outlined above, we believe we approach core factors such as fidelity, dissemination, and sustainability differently than other more rigid approaches.

Fidelity

Program developers sometimes indicate that adhering to original program content, structure, and facilitation is absolutely required and no deviation is allowed. That is, many programs are scripted in their delivery and facilitators are required to follow curriculum guides to the tee. Every facilitator who ever provides a program is supposed to deliver it in the exact same way every time. In TA train-the-trainer programs, we provide a logic model, manuals and checklist reviewing key fidelity guidelines, pre-and-post session rating scales, and require that facilitators practice delivering modules in front of their peers and receive systematic feedback using structured rating forms. We also use a "fishbowl" method in which new facilitators observe a master trainer deliver the program to a group of outside participants and then debrief. We define a master-level trainer as someone who has completed initial certification of the training-of-trainers, has taught several classes, provides evidence of pre-to-post effectiveness, and is certified by the lead author or another master-level trainer.

These methods provide clear guidance for fidelity. However, following the meta-theory tension between fidelity and adaptation (see Figure 15.4), TA also encourages adaptability in three-ways: (a) discovery is built into the curriculum itself (i.e., use of focus groups, investigate local resources and risks); (b) facilitators are trained to personalize some content; and (c) key learning themes, language, and branding should be customized to local conditions. Focus groups and discovery (e.g., learning about local policy, human resources, occupational risks) are built into the intervention process as a preliminary step. For example, policy information (Module 2), tolerance scenarios (Module 3), and NUDGE case studies (Module 6) are modified to fit local policies, occupation and job type, and any risks identified through discovery.

Facilitators are trained to touch upon key elements so participants receive the same overarching information. However, we have found through satisfaction and session ratings that TA, and subsequent adaptations, have been *most impactful* (e.g., greatest improvement in outcomes from pre to-post intervention) when facilitators are sensitive to the population being served and they incorporate their own experiences into the training. In train-the-trainers, where a master-level trainer trains facilitators, we encourage new facilitators to share their own history (e.g., on recovery, resilience, seeking help). Doing so fosters psychological safety in the training environment and, when appropriate, encourages self-disclosure amongst participants.

Accordingly, our fidelity guidelines do not require facilitators to read from a script. Rather, we provide a main set of objectives, important examples, activities, and necessary information in bullet points. Facilitators should feel confident about what is required for participants to understand the content. They can personalize information and empower participants to apply that information to their own personal situation. Participants are more likely to share their own experiences, retain information and skills, and enjoy the experience more when the facilitator tailors examples to their own experiences. In broad adaptations for distinct populations, we create more comprehensive modifications. For example, with *Team Resilience*, we learned that young restaurant workers were more interested in sharing stories with each other about their personal resilience—getting through tough times—and feeling heard. They wanted and needed much less information about policy. Accordingly, we created a new resilience framework to guide their discussions. These "Five Cs of Resilience" (Confidence Commitment, Centering, Community, and Compassion) have been incorporated into a number of corporate programs and e-learning (Bennett et al., 2018).

When adapting the TA curriculum for use in the National Guard, the name of the program was changed to Team *Readiness*, with readiness a familiar term used across all branches of the military. Team Readiness was adapted throughout the program by changing verbiage to reflect typical language used in the military; these changes contributed to the perceived face validity and "buy-in" but did not affect core objectives. Also, the military population was gravely concerned about suicide risk amongst service members returning from Iraq/ Afghanistan. For this reason, the module on stress was expanded into several modules that placed more emphasis on recognizing and getting help for PTSD.

Dissemination and Sustainability

To help promote dissemination, the original TA curriculum (slides, facilitator notes, and manual of the full program) was made available at no cost to the public and online through the IBR and OWLS websites. Evidence-based online registries provided links to these websites so that the curriculum was downloadable to potential providers (e.g., non-profit and community organizations). Until recently, this dissemination method was mostly passive. We waited for individuals, organizations, and institutions to contact us. Between 2002 and 2015 we estimate that close to 1,000 professionals and students (many outside the United States) downloaded the curriculum. We are unsure how many of these individuals actually utilized the curriculum in workplace settings. Many downloads may have been academic in nature.

Even if not used as intended, downloaded materials can be valuable in a variety of ways. They can give potential users a "taste" of the model so they can determine whether it is a good fit for their system or organization and then contact us for consultation and adaptation assistance. They can make some adaptations themselves or pick components or ideas from the curriculum to incorporate in existing or new programs.

Since 2010 we have made concerted efforts to disseminate TA through social media, newsletters, word-of-mouth, and a website. The most frequently used versions of TA are smaller, more digestible modules. While companies do not have the bandwidth for the full cultural intervention represented by the original TA (and its emphasis on substance misuse), users are frequently more ready and interested in addressing stress and wellness. Accordingly, Dr. Bennett authored a book on resilience (Bennett, 2014), we updated Module 4 on stress, and now deliver an on-line webinar-based training of trainers on a regular basis (labeled "Resilience and Thriving").

Sustainability is an evolutionary process, not a destination. Returning to the Integral Model (see Figure 15.4—right side), we learned that being too focused on fidelity in dissemination (requiring strict adherence to manuals and slides) might stymie uptake of the program. Instead, consultation, capacity building, and adaptation tend to facilitate greater diffusion. This chapter began with an example of a case study where we built the TA program for workplace substance use prevention. This particular curriculum was twice reviewed and deemed effective in the National Registry of Evidence-Based Programs and Practices and also in the US Surgeon General's report "Facing Addiction in America" (Office of Surgeon General, 2016). Several iterations of the original program showed us that the best sustainability plan *in our case* was adaptation of content through capacity building.

Lessons Learned and General Advice

In the past 10 years, the OWLS team has used the basic curriculum-development and consultation processes described above to develop or customize trainings for a variety of community-based, government, and corporate clients, from small operations to global businesses. We have used the curriculum-development and consultation more broadly. Those seeking to develop and disseminate *any* prevention program could also use the five-step model and Integral theory. Our experience across these efforts reveals there is no "one size fits all" approach to developing an effective culture of health program.

To stay relevant, workplace prevention curricula must adapt to changes in culture, technology, markets, industries, and the needs of different clients. The original TA curriculum emerged from a grant-funded project for municipal workers and was later promoted through evidence-based registries. These registries have been decommissioned or reorganized, leading us to be more proactive about TA dissemination moving forward. Based on our experience guiding the evolution of TA, this chapter highlighted insights learned from fundamental and seminal processes of development (see Figures 15.1 and 15.2) and later adaptation (see Figure 15.4) that we hope are universally applicable for future preventionists.

References

Bennett, J. (2014). *Raw coping power: From stress to thriving (in life and business)*. Fort Worth, TX: Organizational Wellness & Learning Systems.

Bennett, J. B. (2018). Integral Organizational Wellness: An evidence-based model of socially inspired well-being. *Journal of Applied Biobehavioral Research, 23*(4), e12136.

Bennett, J. B., Aden, C. A., Broome, K., Mitchell, K., & Rigdon, W. D. (2010). Team resilience for young restaurant workers: Research-to-practice adaptation and assessment. *Journal of Occupational Health Psychology, 15*(3), 223–236. doi: 10.1037/a0019379

Bennett, J. B., Cook, R. F., & Pelletier, K. R. (2011). Toward an integrated framework for comprehensive organizational wellness: Concepts, practices, and research in workplace health promotion. In J. C. Quick & L. E. Tetrick (Eds.), *Handbook of occupational health psychology* (2nd ed., pp. 95–118). American Psychological Association.

Bennett, J. B., & Lehman, W. E. (2001). Workplace substance use prevention and help seeking: Comparing team-oriented and informational training. *Journal of Occupational Health Psychology, 6*(3), 243–254. doi: 10.1037/1076-8998.6.3.243

Bennett, J. B., & Lehman, W. E. (2002). Supervisor tolerance-responsiveness to substance use and workplace prevention training: Use of a cognitive mapping tool. *Health Education Research, 17*(1), 27–42. doi: 10.1093/her/17.1.27

Bennett, J. B., Lehman, W. E., & Reynolds, G. S. (2000). Team awareness for workplace substance use prevention: The empirical and conceptual development of a training program. *Prevention Science, 1*(3), 157–172. doi: 10.1023/A:1010025306547

Bennett, J. B., Lucas, G. M., Linde, B. D., Neeper, M. A., Hudson, M., & Gatchel, R. J. (2018). A process model of health consciousness: Its application to the prevention of workplace prescription drug misuse. *Journal of Applied Biobehavioral Research, 23*(3), e12130.

Bennett, J. B., Neeper, M., Linde, B. D., Lucas, G. M., & Simone, L. (2018). Team resilience training in the workplace: E-learning adaptation, measurement model, and two pilot studies. *JMIR mental health, 5*(2), e35.

Bennett, J. B., Patterson, C. R., Reynolds, G. S., Wiitala, W. L., & Lehman, W. E. (2004). Team awareness, problem drinking, and drinking climate: Workplace social health promotion in a policy context. *American Journal of Health Promotion, 19*(2), 103–113.

Bennett, J. B., Reynolds, G. S., & Lehman, W. E. K. (2003, March). The "black box" of health promotion: Employee training-room behaviors predict outcomes. Poster presented at the National Institute on Occupational Safety and Health's Work, Stress, & Health, 2003: Fifth Interdisciplinary Conference on Work Stress, Toronto, Ontario.

Bhatt, D. L., & Mehta, C. (2016). Adaptive designs for clinical trials. *New England Journal of Medicine, 375*(1), 65–74.

Broad, M. L., & Newstrom, J. W. (1992). *Transfer of training: Action-packed strategies to ensure high payoff from training investments.* Reading, MA: Corporate and Professional Publishing Group, Addison-Wesley Publishing Co.

Burnhams, N. H., London, L., Laubscher, R., Nel, E., & Parry, C. (2015). Results of a cluster randomised controlled trial to reduce risky use of alcohol, alcohol-related HIV risks and improve help-seeking behaviour among safety and security employees in the western cape, South Africa. *Substance Use Treatment, Prevention, and Policy, 10*(1), 18–18. doi: 10.1186/s13011-015-0014-5

Cadiz, D. M., O'Neill, C., Butell, S. S., Epeneter, B. J., & Basin, B. (2012). Quasi-experimental evaluation of a substance use awareness educational intervention for nursing students. *The Journal of Nursing Education, 51*(7), 411–415. doi: 10.3928/01484834-20120515-02.

Charmaz, K., & Belgrave, L. L. (2007). Grounded theory. In G. Ritzer (ed.) *The Blackwell encyclopedia of sociology.* Vol. 1479. New York, NY: Blackwell Publishing

Collins, L. M., Murphy, S. A., & Bierman, K. L. (2004). A conceptual framework for adaptive preventive interventions. *Prevention Science, 5*(3), 185–196.

Cook, R. (1985). The alternatives approach revisited: A biopsychological model and guidelines for application. *International Journal of the Addictions, 20*(9), 1399–1419.

Cook, R. F., Back, A. S., & Trudeau, J. (1996). Preventing alcohol use problems among blue-collar workers: A field test of the working people program. *Substance Use and Misuse, 31*(3), 255–275.

Durlak, J. A. (1998). Common risk and protective factors in successful prevention programs. *American Journal of Orthopsychiatry, 68*(4), 512–520.

Edmondson, A. (1999). Psychological safety and learning behavior in work teams. *Administrative science quarterly, 44*(2), 350–383.

Egan, G. (1973). *Face to face: The small group experience.* Publishing, 176. Monterey, CA: Brookes/Cole.

Gelmi, G., Vimercati, N., Celata, C. (2017). Lavoro, Salute, Benessere: Adottare E Adattare Il Programma Team Awareness In Lombardia. In La Psicologia come Scienza della Salute : pre-atti del XII Congresso Nazionale Associazione S.I.P.S.A. Società Italiana di Psicologia della Salute : firenze, 3-5 Novembre 2017 / a cura di Silvia Casale e Amanda Nerini. – Firenze: Firenze University Press, 2017. (Proceedings e report: 116)

Gould, M., Cross, W., Pisani, A., Munfakh, M., & Kleinman, M. (2013). Impact of Applied Suicide Intervention Skills Training on the National Suicide Prevention Lifeline. *Suicide and Life-Threatening Behavior, 43*(6), 676–691. doi: 10.1111/sltb.12049

Holcom, M. L., Lehman, W. E., & Lord, C. G. (1993). Social categorization and the influence of drug involvement on drug attitude structures: Implications for assessing drug use and tolerance in the workplace 1. *Journal of Applied Social Psychology, 23*(23), 1968–1988.

Miller, W. L., Rubinstein, E. B., Howard, J., & Crabtree, B. F. (2019). Shifting implementation science theory to empower primary care practices. *The Annals of Family Medicine, 17*(3), 250–256.

Normand, J., Lempert, R. O., & O'Brien, C. P. (1994). *Under the influence? Drugs and the American work force.* Washington, DC: National Academy Press.

Office of the Surgeon General (2016). Facing addiction in America: The Surgeon General's report on alcohol, drugs, and health. Washington, DC: US Dept of Health and Human Services. Retrieved from http://addiction.surgeongeneral.gov

Patterson, C. R., Bennett, J. B., & Wiitala, W. L. (2005). Healthy and unhealthy stress unwinding: Promoting health in small businesses. *Journal of Business and Psychology, 20*(2), 221–247. doi: 10.1007/s10869-005-8261-5

Petree, R. D., Broome, K. M., & Bennett, J. B. (2012). Exploring and reducing stress in young restaurant workers: Results of a randomized field trial. *American Journal of Health Promotion, 26*(4), 217–224. doi: 10.4278/ajhp.091001-QUAN-321

Reynolds, G. S., & Bennett, J. B. (2015). A cluster randomized trial of alcohol prevention in small businesses: A cascade model of help seeking and risk reduction. *American Journal of Health Promotion, 29*(3), 182–191. doi: 10.4278/ajhp.121212-QUAN-600

Robinson, S. L., & Kraatz, M. S. (1998). Constructing the reality of normative behavior: The use of neutralization strategies by organizational deviants. In R. W. Griffin, A. O'Leary-Kelly, & J. M. Collins (Eds.), *Monographs in organizational behavior and industrial relations, vol. 23, Parts, A & B. Dysfunctional behavior in organizations: Violent and deviant behavior* (pp. 203–220). Stamford, CT: Elsevier Science/JAI Press.

Rollnick, S., & Miller, W. R. (1995). What is motivational interviewing? *Behavioural and Cognitive Psychotherapy, 23*(4), 325–334.

Roman, P. M. (Ed.) (1990). *Alcohol problem intervention in the workplace: Employee assistance programs and strategic alternatives.* Westport, CT: Greenwood Publishing Group.

Schaef, A. W. (1986). *Co-dependence: Misunderstood-mistreated.* San Francisco, CA: Harper & Row.

Small, S. A., Cooney, S. M., & O'connor, C. (2009). Evidence-informed program improvement: Using principles of effectiveness to enhance the quality and impact of family-based prevention programs. *Family Relations, 58*(1), 1–13.

Sonnenstuhl, W. (1990). Help-seeking and helping processes within the workplace: Assisting alcoholic and other troubled employees. In P.M. Roman (Ed.) (1990). *Alcohol problem intervention in the workplace: Employee assistance programs and strategic alternatives.* 237–259. Westport, CT: Greenwood Publishing Group.

Sonnenstuhl, W. J. (1982). Understanding EAP self-referral: Toward a social network approach. *Contemp. Drug Probs , 11*, 269.

Trice, H. M., & Beyer, J. M. (1984). Work-related outcomes of the constructive-confrontation strategy in a job-based alcoholism program. *Journal of Studies on Alcohol, 45*(5), 393–404.

Trice, H. M., & Sonnenstuhl, W. J. (1990). On the construction of drinking norms in work organizations. *Journal of Studies on Alcohol, 51*(3), 201–220.

Index

For Product Safety Concerns and Information please contact our EU
representative GPSR@taylorandfrancis.com
Taylor & Francis Verlag GmbH, Kaufingerstraße 24, 80331 München, Germany

www.ingramcontent.com/pod-product-compliance
Lightning Source LLC
Chambersburg PA
CBHW060353220326
41598CB00023B/2912